# THE POWERLIFTING HANDBOOK

*Practical Principles for Crushing PRs*

# CONTENTS

## Philosophy and Overview

You're about to learn how to become stronger—a lot stronger. To reach your full potential as an athlete, and a human being, building optimal levels of strength is necessary. That's the basis of *The Powerlifting Handbook*—developing levels of strength that give you an edge over your competition, the ability to build the body that you want and the training balance to keep you healthy. Physical success is based upon absolute physical strength.

I outlined many reasons why this is the case in my previous book, *Powerlifitng for the People*. Powerlifting for the People explained exactly why strength is important for all different types of populations and *The Powerlifting Handbook* will teach you the principles it's going to take to get it down and smash new Personal Records (PRs). Because no matter what your goal is and what you are utilizing powerlifting for hitting PRs is what it's all about. Becoming a stronger version of yourself inside and out!

**So, what is absolute strength?**

It is the maximal amount of tension that the muscles can produce against an external load.

As you read, you'll also see me refer to it as maximal strength or limit strength. It's most important to improve maximal strength without a gain in bodyweight. This is known as maximal relative strength.

## Why Strength is King

If you are an athlete, all other attributes being held constant, a stronger athlete is a better athlete. The funny thing about it is that all other physical attributes (such as, speed, power, endurance, etc.) are all direct derivatives of absolute strength. Be you a distance runner, football player or wrestler—developing higher levels of absolute strength will make you a better athlete, and potentially, better at your sport.

Being stronger makes everything easier. Whether it's walking to your car or sprinting to make a tackle—if you are stronger you will expend less energy completing any task.

Consider what researchers found when they studied a group of fifteen female cross-country skiers that trained for maximal upper-body strength for nine weeks.

Compared to the control group in the study, the group of women that trained for maximal upper-body strength increased their absolute strength by a significant margin. That isn't mind blowing. What is mind blowing, however, is the fact that the maximal strength group also improved their time to exhaustion during ergometer testing—by seven minutes (1)! Each turn of the ergometer got a little bit easier because their muscles didn't have to work as hard—showing that improvements in absolute strength have a dramatic effect on over-all muscular endurance.

So, even if you are a middle - aged woman just looking to run your first 5K or mud run getting stronger can help even though you are preparing for an endurance event and not a strength competition.

## Powerlifting for Athletics

Let's take a look at maximum strength for endurance athletes from a different angle—the perspective of a long-distance runner.

Distance runners run for miles at a time—accruing a high number of foot contacts every time that they train and compete. Between each foot contact is a stride that is the product of leg drive. The amount of leg drive a runner has is a direct result of absolute strength—meaning more leg drive equals more distance covered with each stride. Considering the amount of strides made during every run, this can drastically reduce energy expenditure during a race—giving a runner a leg up on the competition. Yes, pun is intended.

Not quite as surprising as absolute strength's effect on endurance is its effect on power. But power is a direct product of absolute strength—without higher levels of maximum strength you will not generate more power (power is force (strength) x velocity (speed)). In the eyes of most coaches, power is the most important physical attribute in predicting athletic success. Sprinting speed and vertical jumping ability are two commonly used measures of power. Absolute strength has proven to be a reliable predictor of performance during both tests.

So, whether you are a competitive athlete or just want to perform a little better in a recreational sport like softball or beach volleyball strength training can help you perform and move better.

When studied using a group of elite, European soccer players—maximum strength in the half-squat was an accurate predictor of both vertical jumping ability and sprinting speed. Seventeen athletes were studied in all and those with the highest one rep max half-squat performed the best on the vertical jump, ten meter sprint and thirty meter sprint (4). The moral of the story—if you can generate more force you'll be more explosive.

Strength training also has a big impact on combat and contact sports. Many men and woman have taken up recreational mixed martial arts and adding strength can certainly help their cause.

Sports like wrestling and football are prime examples of the importance of strength and power. Both sports require violent hip extensions and pulling power to dominate the opposition. In wresting, these actions are needed during the take down—while in football, tackling requires a violent pull and hip extension. Emphasizing deadlift training is important for training the pulling power needed to be a dominating offensive wrestler and defensive football player. Improving absolute strength through the deadlift pattern improves power during hip extension and full-body pulling. Absolute strength breeds power and power breeds domination. The importance of strength cannot be denied.

Science shows us that strength is the king—as evidenced by the two studies above, a stronger body is better able to meet the demands imposed upon it, regardless if the event is based on power or endurance. While training to develop other physical qualities such as power and muscular endurance, are important, training for absolute strength must take precedent—being held almost to the same importance as sport specific skill training.

*I'd* love to tell you that I was the first to adopt the strength first philosophy, but that would be a bold-faced lie. It was, in fact, George Hackenschmidt, the Russian Lion, talked about the importance of strength in his manifesto, *the Way to Live in Health and Physical Fitness,* that he wrote in 1941. Mr. Hackenschmidt wrote, "For it is *only* by exercising with heavy weights that any man can hope to develop really great strength." He continues, "…unless he sedulously carries out the barbell and dumbbell exercises as well, he can never acquire really great physical powers."

These words come from a man who accomplished feats of strength and ruled his competition. In a world before strength was popular, Hackenschmidt trained with unrivaled vigor—accomplishing a 365 pound bench press from the back bridge position. His strength carried over to his career as a wrestler. Hackenschmidt wrestled 3000 matches in his storied career—he lost only two.

Since the days of Hackenschmidt, there have been millions of iron disciples that have spread the good word about strength and they have made the sports world a better place. Because of them, female soccer players hoist barbells and marathon runners push the limits of their maximal strength. For this, I am grateful.

## Powerlifting for Powerlifting

The principles outlined in this book are going to get you stronger. If you apply these principles correctly, you will be hitting PRs for many years to come. If you are powerlifting with the goal to eventually compete these principles hold even more weight since the exercises you will be performing are the lifts you will need to master in order to achieve a better total in competition. That being said EVEN if you goal ISN'T to compete and you simple want to get stronger these methods and principles have been proven work for those just starting out and have also helped mold many nationally ranked lifters and even one best in the world at our little garage gym in Farmingdale NY.

The better understanding you have of these principles, the more you will get out of your training while remaining injury free. Even though powerlifting is a test of absolute strength your mindset should be that of a marathon not a sprint. Slow and steady wins the race. You don't want to burn out by doing too much work too soon. Slow steady gains over time will always trump a big spike in performance followed by a burnout. This will allow you to compete in your sports for many years while making progress. At the time of writing, I am in my 10th competitive year and I am still making progress. I owe much of my knowledge to one man in particular.

# WESTSIDE CONJUGATE METHOD (WCM)

Conversations about the classic men of strength and sports training commonly include names such as Siff, Zatsiorsky, Hackenschmidt, and Vasily Alexseyev. Mel Siff and Vladimir Zatsiorsky have gone to great lengths to improve understanding of strength science. Hackenschmidt and Alexseyev have shown the world what feats of strength mortal men are capable. Whether through science or practice—these men have laid the foundation upon which a castle of strength and power is built. Although impressive, this castle looks much more like a weight-room; and rather than being in some fabled British Isle, it's actually in Ohio.

Many have spread the good word of strength and its positive effect on health and athletic performance, but one man in Ohio has done more for strength than any other. Louie Simmons and his group of powerlifters at Westside Barbell have set the strength precedent. In a world full of mixed up training philosophies based on trends and fads, Mr. Simmons developed the Westside Conjugate Method (WCM) using science, experience, blood, sweat, and chalk.

As is the case for strength coaches all over the world, Louie Simmons and his WCM have had an immeasurable impact on my coaching philosophies and, subsequently, the *Powerlifting Handbook*. The fact that I am still a competitive powerlifter accentuates Westside's impact on my training because I have felt, personally, the effects of conjugate style training at its finest. I know first-hand the dramatic effect that developing maximal strength has on health and athletic performance.

My experience as an athlete and as a coach inspired me to borrow from the components of the WCM in developing *all of my programs at Gaglione Strength*—lift heavy, lift fast and lift for reps. These ideas encompass the maximum effort method, submaximal effort method, dynamic effort method and the repetition effort method. They are the main components that many athletes and powerlifters—disciples of Louie Simmons—have used to develop Simmons—have used to develop their physical prowess. Moreover, as we have learned them, we now extend them to you.

Good training programs are based on periodization. Periodization is essentially how you organize your training. As the late Dr. Mel C. Siff defined it, periodization is, "…a method of alternating training loads to produce peak performance for a specific competitive event." It allows for training variables to be manipulated systematically, producing gains in physical strength and athleticism. In the West, periodization traditionally follows a linear progression—starting with a high volume block of training and progressing down to lower volume training with higher intensity. Following this format, athletes only work to develop one quality at a time (endurance, hypertrophy, strength, and power). This isn't the case with conjugate periodization.

Conjugate literally means "joined together; coupled." Therefore, with conjugate periodization, training is planned to develop multiple qualities at once—rather than working on one physical quality at a time. This creates a training environment that is more closely related to sport—as strength, power and muscular endurance are all needed in sport concurrently. Conjugate periodization also produces gains that are more consistent and sustainable when compared with linear periodization. During linear periodization, the initial gains in endurance and muscular hypertrophy are lost by the time an athlete reaches the power phase of the program. However, conjugate periodization allows for smaller, more sustainable gains in strength, power, hypertrophy, and muscular endurance.

The conjugate method first grew out of the training methods developed at the Dynamo Club in what used to be the Soviet Union. After years of experimentation, Louie Simmons constructed the WCM by combining Bulgarian style maximum effort training and the conjugate training of the former Soviet Union. The resulting philosophy has changed the way powerlifters, athletes and fitness enthusiasts around the world train.

The WCM, and all strength training, is comprised of three main methods of training: maximum effort, dynamic effort, and repetition effort (as well as a few smaller ones). I have outlined them for you below, as they comprise nuts and bolts of *The Powerlifting Handbook*.

## PRINCIPLES OF POWERLIFTING

**Maximum Effort Method:**

Louie Simmons defines the max effort method as lifting a maximal load against maximal resistance. He adapted the idea from the training methods of Bulgarian weightlifting—which involves working to a maximum effort daily on a given lift (usually the squat) (3).

Most lifters, and athletes with weight-room experience, are familiar with the idea of "maxing out," the process by which a one repetition maximum is determined for a given lift. The Maximum Effort (max effort) Method is based on a continuous cycle of working to a five, three or one repetition maximum for a given lift.

Essentially, you are maxing out every week and exercises are rotated regularly to avoid nervous system burnout.

As an example, instead of working to a five, three or one rep maximum every week on the bench—bench press variations are cycled from week to week, month to month or cycle to cycle. You can continually train with heavy weights—making your nervous system more efficient—without hindering your recovery and eventually regressing.

This is the main difference between what we do at Gaglione Strength and what is typically thought of using the WCM is that we aren't doing true maximum effort single at or above 90% all the time. We utilize the Max Effort Method at specific times in our training cycles, in order to test out our lifters limit strength. For example earlier in the training cycle we might test out a 5RM and then, later a 3RM and eventually take some heavy singles toward the end of the training block.

This allows us to have markers along the way to see if the lifter is making progress without truly maxing out all of the time. Typically, when doing max effort training more equipment is used for support. For example: a raw classic lifter will use tight knee sleeves, wrist wraps, and a tight belt for squatting. An equipped lifter would use knees wraps and a squat suit in addition to the previous items mentioned. When you utilize the maximum effort method you want maximum support!

**Max Effort Guidelines**

Typically, it is just one all out set doing minimal warm ups only as need so you can go all out on your primary working set and really test out where you are at.

For example if you are taking a 5Rm your last warm up could be a double or triple near the weight you are going to try. 3RM your last warm up could be a single or double near the weight you are going to try to conserve your energy. When going for a new ....

8Rm you will typically use around 77-80% of your 1RM if you hit more than that percent that is a good indication your 1RM is going up.

5RM you will typically use around 85-87.5% of your 1RM if you hit more than that percent that is a good indication your 1RM is going up.

3Rm you will typically use around 90-93% of your 1RM if you hit more than that percent that is a good indication your 1RM is going up.

The higher percent and closer you are to your previous 1RM the best chance of carry over your will get when you actually test your 1RM or compete in a meet. So a 3Rm is a much better indicator of strength than an 8RM for example. It is closer to what you are actually going to do in a competition.

## Dynamic Effort Method:

Be you an athlete, lifter, or gym rat—there is no denying the dramatic effect that speed and power have on performance. The dynamic effort method is designed to enhance both. Like the submaximal effort method, the dynamic effort method employs submaximal weights— the difference being that the concentration is on generating the maximum amount of speed with every rep during dynamic effort training. This is also known as rate of force development.

Dynamic effort training was introduced to the WCM method to compliment the max effort training days. While traditional Bulgarian training has a lifter work to a max effort every day during training (sometimes multiple times within the same day), Louie Simmons saw that this was having a detrimental effect on the recovery of some lifters. After a stall in his own training—feeling strong but slow—Simmons started to implement the dynamic effort method (2).

Traditional dynamic effort training is done with loads between forty and sixty percent; using eight or nine sets of three on the bench, ten to twelve sets of two for the squat, and six to ten sets of one for the deadlift—usually with some kind of accommodating resistance (bands or chains). The more accommodating resistance you use the lower % of your 1RM is required.

Why is using bands and chains important for speed work? It accommodates the strength curve. The band tension is highest at the lockout portion or the lift and the chain weight is fully loaded at the lockout as well. During the bottom, the bands have the least tension and the chains are fully de-loaded on the ground. If the athlete doesn't lift the first explosively they will slow down or worse, get stuck. This teaches the lifter to lift fast and push through sticking points. It allows for the greatest amount of force production with a lower weight. Typically a lower 1RM would required less chain weight and band tension and a higher 1RM would warrant more chain weight and band tension. One chain per side or a mini band would be perfectly fine for a novice lifter where as a more advanced athlete may use two to three chains per side or light bands or average for dynamic work.

Most people get too carried away with using too much accommodating resistance too early in their training career.

I suggest learning how to set up chains and bands from a qualified coach for this reason.

With this method you can essentially turn any barbell lift (with in reason) into power exercise. Olympic lifting for example is know for developing great power in athletes can be very difficult to learn proper form. When proper form isn't utilized there can be a great risk for injury.

Dynamic effort training with the bench squat and deadlift in addition to jumps and medicine ball throws are great alternative for athletes to use to develop power with a much lower learning curve and less chance for injury. Wrists, hands and elbows typically take a beating when learning Olympic lifts so substitutes speed deadlifts and jumps for power cleans and snatches can be a great alternative for an athlete looking to get more explosive. This doesn't mean weight lifting doesn't have its place in an athletes training as it should all be about risk and reward. It is just important to weight all of your options and powerlifting with the dynamic effort method is an awesome option for a wide variety of athletes.

Another benefit of dynamic effort training is technique practice. For example if you do 3x8 at 60% in the squat it is the exact same volume as 8x3 in the squat at 60% BUT in the second example using the dynamic effort method you get 8 first repetitions versus only three first repetitions in the first example.

When doing a high amount of sets and lower amount of reps you can build a lot for volume with quality repetitions. You get many opportunities to practice your set up and really dial in your technique. In a powerlifting contest the first rep is what you get judged on so it has a better transfer to sport practice then grinding out high rep sets where you only get a few first reps.

Typically, on dynamic days, minimal gear is used. A loose belt and wrist wraps is typically all that is needed. Early in a training cycle beltless work can be used as well as lower percent.

## Dynamic Training Considerations

### Straight Weight

For straight weight dynamic work typically 6-12 sets of 1-3 reps are used with 70%-80% of the lifters 1RM

For example, 8 sets of 2 reps at 70% of 1RM for the squat
For a lifter with a max of 195 that would be 8 sets of 2 at 135.

### Chains
For dynamic work with chains typically 6-12 sets of 1-3 reps are used with 55%-65% of the lifters 1RM

For example 9 sets of 3 reps with 60% of 1RM with one chain per side for the bench

For a lifter with a max bench of 310 that would 185 with 40 lbs of chain (one per side)

### Bands
For dynamic work with band tension typically 6-12 sets of 1-3 reps are used with 40%-50% of the lifters 1RM

For example 8 singles with doubled mini bands for the deadlift

For a 635 deadlifter that would be 315 with about 90 lbs of tension from a slight deficit on a band platform

### Repetition Effort Method:

It's inevitable—you're going to get fatigued. It will happen during training and during competition, so time must be set aside to prepare to perform while tired. You'll also need some gains in muscular hypertrophy to support your gains in strength. Repetition effort training helps build muscular endurance while also promoting hypertrophy gains.

This mode of training entails working to failure—or very close to it. Along with your gains in hypertrophy and muscular endurance, you'll also be challenged—taken to the very brink of what you think you are. As a result, you'll achieve a whole new level of mental toughness.

When you think repetition training you should think to train like "body builder." Body builders are the best at adding muscle so we can all take a few pointers from them. When using body weight movements, cables, bands, or DBs for repetition work you should be really trying to engage your muscles and feel them working.

So if you are doing a triceps exercise for examples really try to engage your triceps during the movement. Don't use a lot of momentum just to get more reps or use more weight. Get a good mind muscle connection and you will get more out of the movement. Remember there is no triceps extension contest at the end of your training cycle! Most likely you are using the triceps extension to assist your bench so just keep that in the back of your head when doing them! Always train with a purpose and understand why you are doing each exercise!

**Repetition Method Considerations**

There are many ways to use the repetition effort method. You can multiple sets of higher reps and go close to failure or to muscular failure. Or you can hit target number of reps and do it in as few sets as possible here are two examples.

Pull - Ups

Get 50 total reps in as few sets as possible

It might look something like this for someone who can do 18-20 pull ups in a row: 12, 11 10, 10, 7

OR they could just try to get 5 sets of 10 reps

You can also do timed sets and really slow down the pace and focus on working the muscle.

For example
For DB bench hit 3 sets of a minute

This will force you pace yourself and really focus on the muscle doing the work versus just using momentum.

In each case you would try to increase the total volume (set times reps) each week in order to progress.

## Submaximal Effort Method:

As the max effort method is used as a main lift for a training session, the submaximal effort method is mainly used during assistance lifts or supplemental exercises. During earlier phases and throughout a training cycle, however, we will use submaximal training to build a base strength level—preparing for the subsequent phases.

The submaximal effort method can be used for any exercise. Applying total volume through prescribing different set and rep schemes is dependent upon the phase of training and the associated goals—as well as upon the nature of the exercise. A general rule to follow is sets of six to eight for strength work, while sets of eight to twelve are used for hypertrophy (muscle growth).

## Submaximal Training and Volume Considerations

One of the biggest mistakes I see when people are doing volume training is them doing volume at too high of an intensity. This can cause the weight to move slow or the lifter to break down in technique. When doing volume training you want to get in as many quality repetitions as possible.

There are many people set and rep schemes for volume training. 5x5 and 3x3 come to mind. Whether you are doing 3 set 5 or 5 sets of 5 or 5 sets of triples here are some general guidelines on how you can approach these types of workouts.

In order to achieve the highest volume without making it a max effort day you can use these percent as general guidelines. These guidelines will make the workouts challenging but still doable.

It is also important to note typically females can handle higher volumes at a higher intensity. This has been shown time and time again by many great female lifters in the world. I first learned about this phenomenon this by former All time Record holder Caitlyn Trout who squatted 391 lbs at being 123 pounds. And typically, people tolerate squatting and benching at higher volumes better than deadlifting in general.

**For multiple sets of 8**
Use around a 12 rep max weight or 65-75% of max

For weaker and female lifters and less sets use closer to 70-75% of max

Example for 3 sets of 8 reps for a 225 squatter might use around 150-160 for working sets

For larger and stronger male lifters use closer to 65-75%% of max

Example a 650 squatter might use 405-435 for 3 sets of 8

**For multiple sets of 5**
Use around a 8RM-10RM weight or 75-80%

For weaker and female lifters and less sets use closer to 80%

Example for 3 sets of 5 reps for a 315 deadlift might use around 245 for working sets

For larger and stronger male lifters use closer to 75%% of max

Example a 500 deadlifter might use 365 for 3 sets of 5

**For multiple sets of 3**

Use around a 5Rm weight or 83-87.5% of max

For weaker and female lifters and less sets use closer to 87.5% of max
A 135 bencher might use 120 for 5 sets of 3 reps

For larger and stronger male lifters use closer to 83% of max

405 Bench might use 335 for 5 sets of 3 reps

By using these guidelines, you are always ensuring you are leaving a few reps in the tank. This is key for progress. You should never be grinding or missing weights on a volume day. If you are using the submaximal effort method on a supplemental lift the percent should be cut even lower by another 10% or so. The main thing is these percent are just guidelines. Always go by feel and make sure you are getting good quality reps in.

When using these guidelines it is important to be aware of the gear you are using when testing your 1RM. For example if you are using a 1RM in tight knee sleeves a tight belt or using knee wraps you need to be more conservative with your % and lower your intensity accordingly. This is why Jim Wendler likes to use 90% of his 1Rm to start his programs. It's a way of starting light so you have a solid chance to build up.

**Other Components and Considerations**

**Improving your Technical Max Versus Absolute Max**

Another approach to doing rep maxing is using a technical max. This is what I recommend to newer lifters. A technical max is the heaviest weight you can do with exceptional form. If your form breaks down the set is over. For example, you might be able to deadlift 405 for a single with perfect form but your max is 495 with round back or with a hitch. 405 is your technical max and 495 if your absolute max. Imagine if that same lifter could get their deadlift to 455 with perfect position. Imagine how much better their attempt will look with 495 the next time they try it. Improving technique at higher weight can make a world of difference. Really accomplished lifters technical max and absolute maxes are very close or even identically.

Most of the time when an elite lifter misses a weight but stay in good position it is do to just fact they are not strong enough even. Sometimes an elite lifter may make they 1RM look effortless because they are in such good position. Whereas a novice lifter 1RM make look awful. You always want to strive to improve your technical max. As your technical max improves so will your absolute max.

This will also allow you to train at higher volumes and intensity because you will be in between position and have a lot less joint stress. A good rule of thumb is when your form breaks down a lot shut it down. Don't do any more weight. Either lower the weight or move on. That will give you the best training effect without any added stress on your joints or body.

## Underloading

Early on in your training cycle, I recommend to utilize movements that are harder so you won't have to use as much bar weight. That way it's easy on joints but a greater stimulus on the muscles.

For example my strong squatting position is low bar with feet wide and flat shoes. I utilized high bar squats and front squats with a narrow stance in heels to build up my legs and back early in my last meet prep training cycle.

My stronger pressing style is a wider grip with my feet back. Early in my meet prep I used a closer grip with my feet up with a longer pause. This allowed me to use slightly lower training weights early on in the cycle while still giving me great stimulus.

As I got closer to peaking I started to go closer and closer to my competition stance and grip. This really helped build my strength while keep stress on my joints really low and allowed my body to recover much quicker.

## *Underloading examples*

*–Front loaded over back loaded*

*Front Squats and Goblet Squat over back squats*

*Belly Swing (front loaded DB) over RDL*

*–More Range of Motion*

*Deficit Deadlifts (standing on a plate) over deadlifts*

*Buffalo Bar Bench (cambered bar with more range) over bench press*

*–Tempo (Isometrics and Eccentrics)*

*Long Pause Bench (pause 3 second on chest) over regular bench*

*Eccentric Front Squat (slow lowering) over Squat*

*Pause Deadlift (pause at knee for 3 seconds) over deadlift*

*–Harder Stance/Grip*
*Narrow Squats and benches over wide squats and bench presses*

*Examples of Underloading workouts*

*Pause Squats using 365 for 3 sets of 8 reps with a 3 second pause and no belt for a 645 squatter*

*Long Pause Bench with Feet Up 245 with wide grip and 3 second pause 5x5 for a 365 bencher*

*Deficit Deadlifts Standing on a 45 pound plate with no belt 405 for 3
sets of 5 for a 635 deadlifter*

## Overloading

Overloading is a technique you can utilize to feel more weight to
stimulant your central nervous system. Essentially you are tricking
your body in to being able to handle heavier weights for a period of
time. This make is perfect during a peak phase as you get closer to a
contest.

At Gaglione Strength we like to use overload training at least once per
training cycle usually the week before we take a heavy single before a
contest or the week before we test our lifts.

For squats and deadlifts, I utilized reverse bands. By using this
technique you will set up giant rubber bands inside of a power rack.
The key is setting up the band so the tension is about zero at the
top so you feel the straight weight that is on the bar. See where you
lockout your lift and adjust the pins accordingly to set up the bands
correctly. Having a qualified coach teach you is always recommend.
I also suggest inspecting bands to make sure they in good condition
before using.

For bench I utilized the sling shot but reverse bands could be used as
well. This is a supported device that that stretches and flexes like the
muscles of your body helping you move weight of your chest put lets
go at lockout so you feel the weight in your hands while reducing the
stress on the shoulder and aiding in the first part of the press.

The main goal here was to simply feel some heavy weight on my back
or in my hands each month. This allowed my nervous system to adjust
even though I was using lighter weights for a good portion of the
training cycle.

If you don't have access to bands utilizing heavy walk outs and unrack
and holds to simply feel the weight for squat and bench are good ideas.

That being said picking up a pair of mini bands will only cost a few dollars and is certainly worth the investment. This will allow you to go through a full range of motion but you still get to feel the straight weight on your back.

We recommend gets bands from elitefts.com and you can also get jump stretch bands from amazon.com, as well. You can purchase a slingshot from howmuchyabench.net.

### *Overload Examples*

*Full Range*
*Reverse Bands for squat, bench, deads and Sling Shot for Bench*

*Partial Range Pin Squats, Pin Presses, Rack Deads*

*Other Considerations*
*Heavy Walk Outs for squats and Unrack and hold for presses*

Examples of Overload Workouts

*Work up to squat opener than reverse mini bands for $2^{nd}$ attempt. Reverse Monster mini band for third attempt*

*Work up to bench opener and bench $2^{nd}$ attempt. Sling Shot bench press $3^{rd}$ attempt for as many reps as possible.*

*Reverse mini band deadlift opener for 3 singles.*

### *Quality over Quantity*

A very quick but important principle. Always leave a little in the tank. Try to go to technical failure instead of muscular failure. This allows for best recovery and also keep you from forming bad habits.

Dan Green refers to this as the technical max. Your technical max is the heaviest weight you can do with perfect form. The absolute max is the heaviest weight you can lift regardless of form.

Elite lifters technical max and absolute max is usually the same or very close where as a beginner lifter the technical max is much less than their absolute max. This could be due to poor technique; the motor pattern isn't grooved yet or just lack of focus. I recommend training within your technical max and save your absolute max when it comes time to test or your lifts in a contest. Success breeds success. Missing lifts in training can cause bad habits as well as mess with your head. If you are always successful in the gym, you will be successful at the meet.

Strength needs to treated like a skill. Just a like a golf swing or baseball throw. The bench squat and deadlift need to be treated like athletic moves and thousands of reps with perfect form need to be performed in order to ingrain proper technique. Eventually the movement will become natural and second nature.

So again in short. Always focus on getting quality work versus a lot of work with crappy form. Quality over quantity. More isn't better, better is better.

## Picking Smart Supplementals

The second barbell lifts or supplemental exercise I choose are specific to my weak points and quite frankly it's what I sucked at. Besides my deadlift my weakness is more bottom end so for squats and bench press I choose exercises that reflected that weak point. If you know you weak point is the lockout you can certainly spend more time training that weakness. Also being a primarily a geared lifter my technique was also a weakness so I picked exercises that helped build my technique as well.

As you get more advanced typically your primary exercise will be the squat bench or deadlift and the second movement will be a variation of the main lift that will aid in your weak point.

*-**Supplemental** Exercises for the Squat*

*Bottom End: Front Squats, Low Box Squats*

*Top End: Anderson Pin Squats, Squats with Chains/bands*

*Technique: Pause Squats*

*-**Supplemental** Exercises for the Bench Press*

*Bottom End: Wide Grip Long Pause Bench with Feet Up, Incline Press*

*Top End: Board/Spotto Presses, Bench with Chains/bands*

*Technique: Long Pause Bench*

*-**Supplemental** Exercises for Deadlift*

*Bottom End: Deficit Deadlift, Stiff Leg*

*Top End: Block Pull, RDL, Deadlifts with chains/bands*

*Technique: Pause Deadlift*

# THE TRAINING DAY

Each day will start with a warm-up; comprised of a soft-tissue improvement technique called self-myofascial release followed by mobility training. From the warm-up, you'll transition into primary exercise and then move on to supplemental and accessory work If you move at the right pace, your training session should last no longer than an hour and a half.

Here is the layout of a good strength training session.

Warm Up
-SMR (Self Myofascial Release)
-Mobility (usually hips, ankles and t-spine)
-Activation (usually core, glutes, and upper back/lats)

Sample Basic Warm Up

A1) Rolling Planks with belly breathing Focus
B1) Band Face Pulls
C1) Band Side Steps
D1) Squat to Stand
E1) Reverse Lunge with Overhead Reach

Strength Workout

-Primary Exercise (squat, bench or deadlift usually)

-Supplemental Exercise (squat, bench, deadlift variation)
-Accessory Exercise (3-5 movement usually isolation or lower level exercises)

Sample Basic Workout

A1) Squat 5x5

B1) 3 Count Pause Squat 3x8

C1) Glute Ham Raise 3x10
C2) Weight Planks 2x:20 seconds
C3) Bulgarian Split Squat 2x12 per side

# THE TRAINING WEEK

Planning your training week is one of the biggest obstacles to overcome for a coach and trainee. Having a plan that ensures that the right training falls on the right day can be as important as the sets, reps and exercises that make up the program. A mismanaged training week will inhibit your recovery from training, making your trips to the weight room about as productive as installing a screen door on a submarine.

We'll be upfront in telling you that lifting four consecutive days while following any program won't work. Plain and simple, it will be too much for your body to handle and you won't recover. We also advise against the two days on, one day off and then two days on training week. You will still be setting your body up for failure, especially during the later phases of the program. It just won't work.

What does work is separating three of your training days with a day of rest in between, then training two days successively. Would you like a visual?

*Monday: Lower-Body (Max Effort)*

*Tuesday: Off (optional conditioning)*

*Wednesday: Upper-Body (Max Effort)*

*Thursday: Off (optional conditioning)*

*Friday: Lower-Body (Dynamic Effort)*

*Saturday: Upper-Body (Dynamic Effort)*

*Sunday: Completely off*

As you'll notice above, putting a day of rest between your max effort training days works best. This day off allows your nervous system to recover. If your nervous system is overloaded with two days of heavy training consecutively—it will tell you to go fly a kite. Group the dynamic effort days and keep the max effort days separated.

For early phases of a program, there are no max effort or dynamic effort training days—the same submaximal effort loads are used for each training session. Since you don't have to worry about separating max effort training days, just make sure that there are two days of rest in the middle of the week. The nervous system won't be taxed quite as much, so you will still be able to recover for the two consecutive training days at the end of the week.

For a three-day program, you can also break it up like this. I used this split with my athletes for many years with great success. It allowed for great recovery when they were doing skill work and they often had competitions on weekend so it worked out really well.

*Monday: Lower-Body (Max Effort)*

*Tuesday: Off (optional conditioning)*

*Wednesday: Upper-Body (Max Effort)*

*Thursday: Off (optional conditioning)*

*Friday: Total-Body (Dynamic Effort)*

*Saturday: Off*

*Sunday: Completely off*

## Another way to break up the week

Over the year, I used the above template with great success. As I started training more and more athletes and I had less and less time for myself I decide to make things a little simpler. Now Max Effort and Dynamic effort methods are sprinkle throughout the work month and each day has a dedicated lift for it. Here is another way of potentially breaking up your training.

*Monday: Lower-Body (Squat Focused)*

*Tuesday: Off (optional conditioning)*

*Wednesday: Upper-Body (Bench Focused)*

*Thursday: Off (optional conditioning)*

*Friday: Lower-Body (Deadlift Focused)*

*Saturday: Upper-Body (Bench Assistance Focused usually incline or overhead press)*

*Sunday: Completely off*

## For training three days a week, another option would be:

*Monday: Lower-Body (Squat Focused)*

*Tuesday: Off (optional conditioning)*

*Wednesday: Upper-Body (Bench Focused)*

*Thursday: Off (optional conditioning)*

*Friday: Lower-Body (Deadlift Focused and Bench Assistance)*

*Saturday: Off*

*Sunday: Completely off*

This is how the majority of my lifters training has been currently. It allows them to hit upper and lower body twice a week during three sessions, which will allow for more recovery and free time for their career and family.

## LOADING PARAMETERS AND PROGRESSIONS

Before starting any program, it's always a good idea to do what I like to call a movement preparation phase. A movement preparation phase could last anywhere from two-six weeks or longer depending on the fitness level of the individual and their personal goals.

Generally, a movement prep phases won't include any barbell movements, mostly body weight and dumbbells to help groove movement patterns and allow the body to handle exercises that are more advanced in later phases. The goal simply to make sure that the body is ready for barbell work.

Seasoned athletes may only need a week or two, but someone who is very deconditioned may need a month or a month and a half to get back in the swing of things.

Each phase—after the movement prep phase—will typically consist of three weeks of training plus a de-load week. The length of each phase is typically one month. Volume loading will be approached in two ways—escalating volume and varying volume.

During initial phases of training the volume will increase each week for the first three weeks—followed by a volume cut on the fourth week during the first de-load.

It's is all about improving the amount of work you do. The overall work for you session is your volume. Essentially, it's your sets times your reps. So, if you did one set of 10 with a 100 lbs, then, you did 1000 lbs of work. If you did two sets of 10 at a 100 lbs you did 2000 lbs of work. That's twice as much volume. Generally do more sets is the best way to increase overall volume over time.

Most beginners can get away with a linear progression for a long time. A person may do an extra set each week or five more pounds. These small progression lead to big gains over time and this is a great way to progress someone new. Slowly increasing the numbers of reps and weights over the course of the training month will help get the body ready for more advanced training methods to come.

Generally beginning phases will feel like hell (because of higher rep ranges and overall volume), but you'll build some great mass and the work capacity necessary to prepare for the next phases of training.

The volume progression for phase one looks like this:

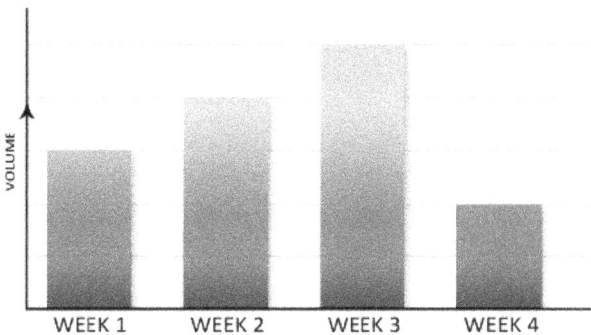

Increasing your volume is a great way to build strength but at some point you will also need to increase intensity as well. Intensity is the percentage of your 1RM. So for example if you are doing 3 sets 3 at 90% of your 1 rep max versus 3 sets of five at 75% of your 1RM the sets at 90% is a higher intensity because it is a heavier load closer to your 1RM. This is where heavy and overload work comes into play.

During later phases two as well during a peaking phase we like to the varying volume loading schedule. Rather than the volume increasing incrementally each week—it loads in a wave.

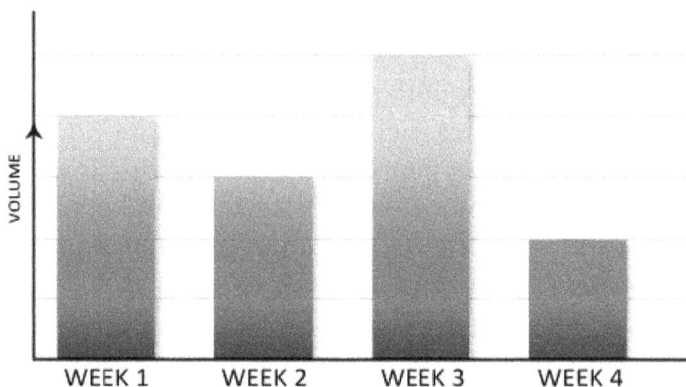

Varying volume loading, also called wave loading, enhances recovery when working at higher intensities of training. And because we will be using principles derived from the WCM method during these phases, optimal recovery will be a must. Making a volume cut during week two of the phase helps with two things. The volume cut will facilitate adaptation to the first week of training while preparing your body for the overreach in volume on week three. De-loading on week four lets your body rest and adapt to the previous three weeks of training. Remember, fatigue masks fitness—de-loading removes fatigue and reveals your true fitness level.

*During a peaking phase, this is especially important. It will allow your body to recovery so you can realize your full potential and display your absolute strength.*

# POWERLIFTING PROGRAM PHASES

Sound training programs are based around well thought-out exercise progressions and training variable manipulations. Each phase of *The Powerlifting Handbook* is designed to progress seamlessly to the subsequent phase—giving your body the chance to adapt to the changes in complexity of movement, workload and intensity. Here is a brief overview of each phase in their programming order. Each phase will be working on different things.

## Movement Prep Phase

Before a movement is heavily loaded, it must be well grooved. For example, you can't expect to deadlift 500 pounds if you aren't hip hinging well. The goal of the movement prep phase is to create balance in your movement in preparation for heavy loading. This phase will last for two weeks for seasoned athletes and lifters—just enough time to move better and improve your work capacity before moving on to bigger weights.

## Phase 1 Building

Max effort training requires an acclimatization period. Initial phases of training are designed to prepare you for max effort training, to improve your work capacity and to build mass in support of your strength gains.

## Phase 2 Strength

Phase 2 introduces the WCM principles. You'll begin max effort training based on movements that are going to help build the bench squat and deadlift. At the end of these secondary phases, you'll begin training full range of motion lifts in your competition stance for max effort. During these secondary phases also marks the beginning of dynamic effort training using the speed variations of lifts such as the bench press, deadlift, box squat, and push press with and without accommodating resistance.

## Phase 3 Peaking

Phase 3 or the peaking phase is designed to develop peak strength. The last month of the program is the culmination of all the work done during the first four phases. Max effort exercises will be done using a full range of motion, and the volume and intensity of the dynamic effort training are both increased. The overload principles will be utilized here to stimulate the central nervous system fully. This will allow the lifter to realize their full potential when it counts. After a de-load week, at the end of the phase, you'll test your progress over the last fourteen weeks.

# Goal Setting

To be strong and successful, you must set clear goals and then hold yourself accountable to achieving them. Self-accountability is dependent upon emotion.

**What Drives You?**

What do I want to change? Why do I want to change it? What outcome(s) do I see in my head?

Ask yourself these three questions before you set any goal. These questions will either reveal your motivation for obtaining a goal, or reveal a proposed goal as a farce. Through the questioning process you'll find what drives you.

Pay special attention to the last question. What do you see in your head? The images should make you feel happy, fulfilled and successful. Hold these images; remember them, because these are what you'll emotionally attach to. These pictures will drive you to achieve your goals.

**Set Your Goals**

After you've asked yourself the above questions, and determined your answers, set your goals. Set a goal for each testing lift and a total outcome for the program. How will achieving your individual goals help you achieve a bigger outcome?

## Write Them Down

After you set your goals—write them down. It doesn't matter what you write on—it could be a dinner napkin. We recommend in your training log and on a scrap piece of paper.

You do, however, need to keep your written goals where you can see them. Keep a copy by your bed so they are the first thing you see in the morning and the last thing you see before you turn out the lights. Look at them and visualize success.

## Taking Action toward Your Goals

Writing your goals down and visualizing success are definitely necessary—this much is true. But all the writing and visualizing in the world won't matter if you don't take action.

Take action every day to achieve your goals. Train hard on your training days, and recover on your off days. Make every step calculated and keep your focus laser tight.

*Here is an example of a goal setting exercise I used on myself many years ago.*

People want to get stronger, leaner, and faster, but oftentimes, they do not have a goal in mind. Let me ask you something, would you go on a trip without a destination? Would you travel somewhere without a map, GPS, or directions? If you do not no where you are going then it is impossible to get better and reach your goals.

In order to get better you need a *PLAN of attack*. You need to write down you goals. By writing down your goals this makes the task real and tangible. Before you write it down the goal is just a thought, an idea a dream. Make the goal real by writing it down and put the goal some place where you can see it every day in order to remind you of what it is you are working on.

Make your goals *specific, measurable, attainable, relevant, and timely*. I will give an example of a goal I had of squatting 675 pounds at my last power lifting meet, but the information in this article can be applied to any goal.

## Specific
I wanted to squat at least 675 (which is 7 plates on each side on a normal 45l b bar). My goal was not to simply squat more, I had a specific number in mind for a specific competition. A person may want to lose 10% body fat or 15 pounds. These are all numbers than can be quantified and measure in a certain amount of time. Specific really entails of the other elements as well.

## Measurable
Make sure the goal is measurable. I wanted to squat 675 at my last powerlifting competition. The way I measure the goal is by going to the meet and getting on the platform in front of three judges. The judges will make sure my form is good and I make good depth. If I don't do a squat according to the rules the lift will not count.
If someone's goal is lose fat, then, they should know how much they want to lose. Numbers and units help us quantify what we are doing. I want to look better is not a good goal, because better is very vague. I want to lose 15 pounds in 3 months is a good goal because it is something we can measure with a scale. Some people may not care how much they weight, but they want a six pack. There will be certain weight and body fat percentage that will give them that look and that number should be their goal.

## Attainable
Goals should be realistic. I squatted 690 in training, but it was a little high and my form was a little off. In a competition if you are a little high the squat will not count. Even though my depth was questionable I was confident that I had the strength to squat at least 675 to proper depth. I also had a plan of attack to reach my goal. I trained with several powerlifters who were better than me. Many of the people I had trained with squatted more than, 700, 800, and even, 900 pounds. I surrounded myself with good people and I got better as a result. I was in a realistic setting for reaching my goal. I was consistently pushing to have better form and work harder each and every workout. The other thing that helped a lot is I saw many people squat in excess of 700

pounds every week so in my brain I knew I could eventually do it too.

The environment you are in is crucial for success. If you want to lose weight you should be around people who support your goals. If you want to become a better wrestler you should wrestle with people who have more experience and better technique than you. People need to get out of their comfort zone and be challenged in order to get better.

## Relevant

Many times, people ask me why do I compete in powerlifting. As an athlete, growing up I always went 100% in every drill and in every training session in order to get better. I learned as an athlete that the harder your work the better you will get, but you also need to work intelligently as well.  Now I am a strength coach and a trainer I want to continue to get stronger and smarter in order to help myself as well as my clients. If I wasn't constantly trying to get stronger why should anyone listen to me about strength. I will constantly push myself  to my body's limit, the same my I expect my athletes and clients to do. I strive to not only "talk the talk" , but more importantly "walk the walk." I want to be a role model for my athletes/clients, inspire them to do better and achieve their goals.

Make sure your goals have meaning to you. Why do you want to get leaner, jump higher, or run faster? Make sure these goals are relevant to your life and have meaning. I know when I played sports I learned many life lessons about team work, work ethic, sacrifice, and goal setting. Training for sports taught me so much about life and helped prepared me for the real world and molded me into a better coach and trainer as a result.

## Timely

Make sure you have a time frame for each goal and set mini goals along the way. I knew in order to squat 675 at some point I would have to squat 600 first, then 650 and so forth. My goal was to squat 675 on August 7th 2010, which goes back to being very specific. Make sure you have enough time to complete your goal and don't be afraid to re-adjust your time frame if you don't make it. Constantly log your progress in order to see if you are approaching your goal. I keep track of my lifts in an exercise journal on my computer to track my progress and to see if I am getting stronger. This also helps me see what assistance exercises are working for me.

If you are trying to get leaner or add muscle keep a food journal (now you can use apps like My Fitness Pal). Keep track of what you're eating. Many times, just by logging the food down will help you eat better since you are more conscious of how much you are eating and what you are eating. You should also weigh yourself once a week at the same time in the same clothes in order to monitor progress for weight change.

I hope these tips will inspire you to have *SMART* goals for the rest of the year. And in case you are wondering, I did get a 675 squat at that particular meet!

# MASTERING THE BASICS

Before embarking on any powerlifting program, there are basics that you need to master. Mastering breathing, bracing and maintaining neutral posture will start you on a path toward success with *The Powerlifting Handbook*. You'll be healthier and stronger for your efforts.

Follow our guide below for taking control of your breathing, learning to brace and maintaining neutral posture while under tension.

## Breathing

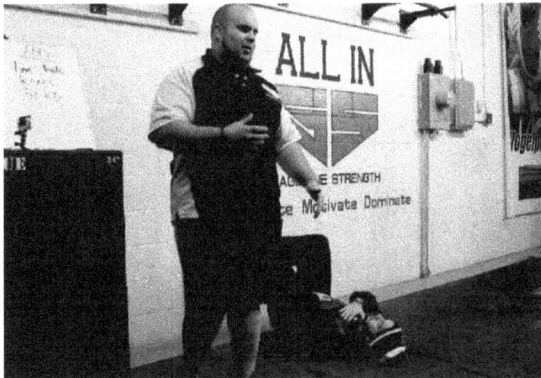

Something during the long lineage of human existence has gotten twisted and people have forgotten how to complete the most fundamental of all movement patterns—breathing. Rather than using our diaphragms to expand our rib cage and take a breath, we incessantly elevate our shoulders and force air higher into our chest cavity. Instead of relaxing and dissipating tension with each breath, we create tension in our upper-trapezius, neck and upper-back.

Incorrect breathing is invasive—disrupting proper movement by creating muscular imbalances that lead to instability throughout the body. It seems like a lot to grasp doesn't it? How could just elevating our shoulders when we breathe cause that much damage? Well, here's an example—courtesy of my good friend Jim Smith of Diesel Strength and Conditioning.

*'Shoulder breathing not only elevates our shoulders, but also extends our lumbar spine—even if only minutely. Over the course of a day those small extensions of the lumbar region can add up, creating anterior pelvic tilt and destabilizing the hips and low-back. Instability at the hips has a ripple effect that can affect joints throughout the body—especially the low-back, shoulders and knees. As serious athletes and lifters, we cannot afford to create instability at these key joints.'*

Good breathing is also the first step of core training. Core stability is developed when the muscles of the inner core and outer core work as a cohesive unit. The diaphragm, the muscles of the pelvic floor and the multifidi are the muscle most commonly associated with the inner core, as they interact to create intra-abdominal pressure.

If coordination between the diaphragm, pelvic floor and multifidi is limited the muscles of the outer core (abdominals, spinal erectors, lats, glutes, etc.) cannot coordinate efficiently.

Coordination of the diaphragm and the pelvic floor begins with solid diaphragmatic breathing. Below we have outlined a breathing progression, adapted from the work of Steve Maxwell, to teach you to breathe again.

**Alligator Breathing**

This drill is called alligator breathing because you will be lying prone (face - down) on the floor, as if you are an alligator. To start, lie on the floor face down with your hands underneath your belly. Make sure that your neck is relaxed and your forehead is resting on the floor. Now, take deep breaths in through your nose and out through your mouth—being sure to transport the air into your belly. If you are doing the drill properly you will feel your belly press out against your hands and into the floor. Alligator breathing should be done for thirty seconds to one minute.

## Supine Belly Breathing

Once alligator breathing is mastered, you will roll over onto your back and work on supine belly breathing. Start by lying supine (face - up) on the floor with your knees bent and your body relaxed. Place your hands on your belly, more specifically, right on your belly button.

As you did during alligator breathing, take deep breaths in through your nose and out through your mouth—transporting the air into your belly. Your belly and, subsequently, your hands should rise with each breath. Once you are breathing solely into your belly, slide your hands to just above your pelvis on each side of your body. Apply pressure there with your fingers to reinforce breathing three dimensionally and filling your entire belly with air. While supine belly breathing, take deep breaths into your belly for thirty seconds to one minute.

## Standing Belly Breathing

Take the skills that you mastered on the floor and transfer them to the upright position. Place your hands on your belly, breathe deeply in through your nose and out through your mouth and transport the air into your belly with each breath—causing your hands to rise. Continue taking deep breaths into your belly for thirty seconds to one minute.

## Walking Breath Ladders

This drill comes directly from the legendary Steve Maxwell. Until now your breathing drills have been done statically and with minimal tension. Now you will walk and belly-breathe at the same time—reinforcing your breath by placing your hands on your belly. Start by inhaling on one step and exhaling on the next step. Next, you'll inhale for two steps and exhale for two steps—followed by inhaling for three steps and exhaling for three steps. The goal is to work up to ten steps while inhaling and ten steps while exhaling and walking at a slow to moderate pace. If you feel as though you are running out of room while inhaling or completely losing all of your air while exhaling—you have included too many steps. Drop back down a few steps and build your lung capacity gradually.

## When to Include Breathing Drills

Breathing drills can be done all the time. You could practice belly breathing before you train, after you train or while you train. An "off day" is a great time to work on belly breathing, and so is while you are watching television or reading. You should be working on reinforcing the belly breathing pattern every day.

## Bracing

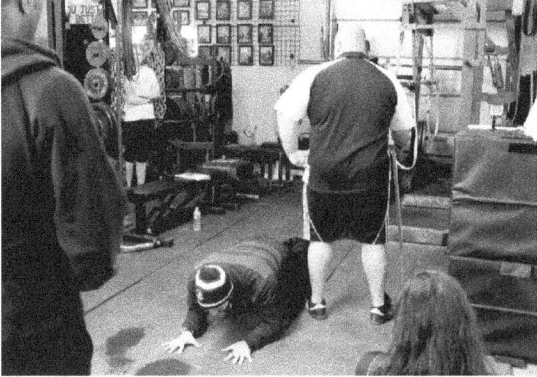

Core strength is based on creating stability—not on doing crunches. Our core is given the dutiful task of protecting our spine as we move in sport and in our daily lives. An isometric co-contraction of the large core muscles, known as bracing, is what gives our core the strength to protect our spine while transferring force between the upper - and lower - body. Let's learn about bracing.

## Air

The section on breathing preceded this section because good breathing patterns are important for bracing. In fact, bracing starts with a good breath of air.

To start a bracing effort, you'll take a deep belly breath—creating the intra-abdominal pressure pivotal for spinal stability. For max effort attempts, or sub-maximal attempts with heavy weight, you will hold your breath after it travels to your belly. For all other movements or isometric holds you will continue deep belly breaths while statically contracting your core musculature. This is known as breathing behind the brace.

## Abs

Bracing requires a powerful abdominal contraction. As you take air into your belly you will tighten your abs forcefully while slightly pushing them out. This begins the core corseting effect by stabilizing the core anteriorly—creating a natural weight-lifting belt. As the abs also attach to the thoracolumbar fascia, it begins the three dimensional bracing effect.

## Lats

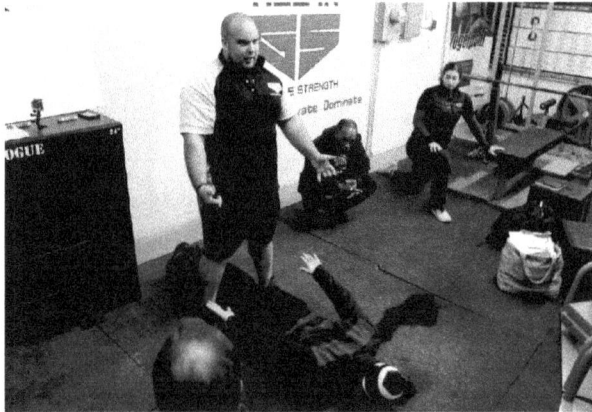

Trainees and coaches often forget about the lats when it comes to creating core stability. But the lats also attach to the thoracolumbar fascia—making them important for bracing and the subsequent corseting effect. While bracing your abs—squeeze your lats tight by depressing your shoulder blades. As you squeeze your lats in succession with your abs, notice that your entire torso becomes rigid and your upper-back pulls into neutral alignment. In addition to bracing your core and aligning your upper-back, you've also created stability in your shoulder girdle. You are one step away from a complete brace.

Having trouble feeling your lats and upper back? Simply lye face down on the floor with your hands near your hips. Lift your hands up and inch of the ground and think about pinching a piece of paper in between your armpits. This is what creating lat tension during the deadlift should feel like.

Do the same drill two more times. Next time, place your hands directly under your elbows. That is what upper back tension for a bench press should feel like. The third time with your elbows bent like you are in the bottom of a pull up or pull down with your thumb up toward the ceiling forming a W shape with your arms. That is what lat tension for a squat should feel like.

**Glutes**

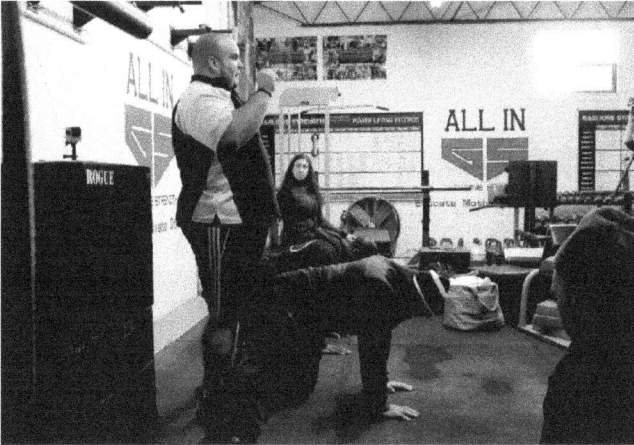

Forcefully contracting your glutes completes the four step bracing process. For upper-body movements, this is an isometric contraction. But for squatting, deadlifting and other lower-body movements, forcefully contract the glutes to create movement.

Tightening and using the glutes ensures stability at the hips. Without a powerful glute contraction, as they are responsible for stabilizing the low-back and neutralizing the pelvis, the muscles of the low-back and hamstrings will be forced to compensate—resulting in a greater injury potential.

Having trouble feeling your glutes? Lie on your back with your legs bent. Drive the hips up toward the ceiling and imagine pinching a coin in between your cheeks. This is what a deadlift lockout should feel like and how your legs should be engaged in a bench (while keeping your butt on the bench of course).

Having trouble feelings your hips? Stand up tall and stamp your feet into the ground with your toes fairly straight ahead. Without changing the direction of your toes think about screwing your feet into the ground and squeezing your glutes. You should feel tension all along the side of your legs. This drill will help keeps your knees out while squatting and sumo deadlifting.

**When to Brace**
You should brace before beginning any exercise—bodyweight or loaded. Let's use the deadlift as an example of how create a good brace.

During your set up, as you approach the bar, take in your breath and tighten your abs. Reach down and grab the bar, then lower your hips and pull your lats tight. Now forcefully contract your glutes as you "push away" from the floor to pull the bar toward lock out. Continue to keep your abs, lats and glutes tight until you finish the lift.

**Creating Tension**

As you brace you will create tension throughout your body. But great amounts of tension start at the points of contact—your feet and your hands.

There are two simple steps to creating high levels of tension. First, grip the bar, dumbbell or other equipment as hard as you can. We call this "melting the bar." Your knuckles should be white, and through a process called irradiation, the muscles of your arm, shoulder girdle and back will subsequently tighten.

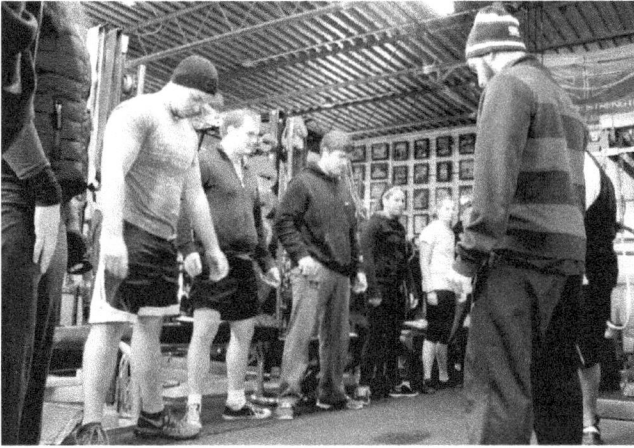

The second way is to create tension in your feet by actively grabbing the floor. You can do this by using your toes like your fingers and squeezing them into the floor. This technique works well for squatting, deadlifting and securing the planted leg during single leg movements. As you felt the muscles of your arms tighten as you set your grip hard with your hands, you'll feel the tension travel up your legs and into your core as you grab the floor with your feet.

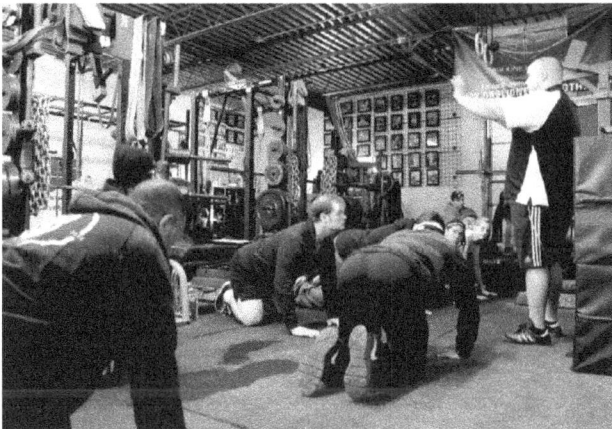

Coordinate tension creation at the points of contact while engaging your brace—this will create full-body stability, improving your ability to demonstrate strength and power.

## Neutral Spine

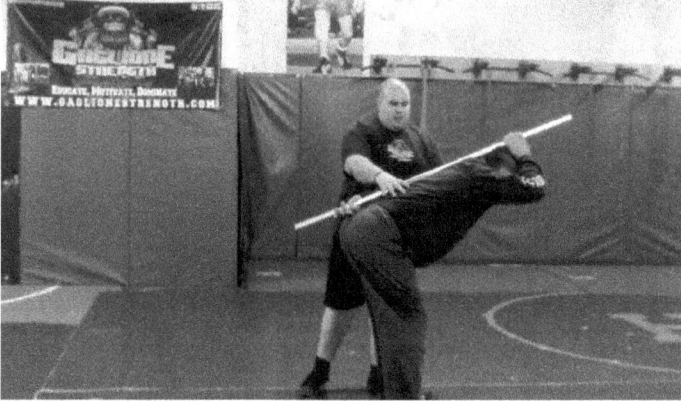

Your goal during any lift should be to maintain neutral positioning of the spine. If your spine is not held in neutral, then you are not stable—and stability is the ultimate goal of strength training.

Training in the neutral position also ensures that you are recruiting muscles with good sequencing—meaning that the right muscles are firing at the right times. This gives us two bits of good news.

First off, good sequencing makes you stronger—and that's our overall goal. But good sequencing also keeps our soft-tissue (muscles, fascia, tendons and ligaments) healthier. As muscles activate in the right pattern the strain of movement is disbursed more evenly through the body—limiting an overload of specific tissues. Maintaining neutral posture of the spine is also important for the alignment of other joints—especially the shoulders and the hips.

Problems at the shoulders and hips that result from poor posture are best described by Dr. Vladimir Janda's Upper- and Lower-Cross Syndromes. Without realizing it, you have seen these misalignments countless times throughout your travels and, possibly, are experiencing them yourself.

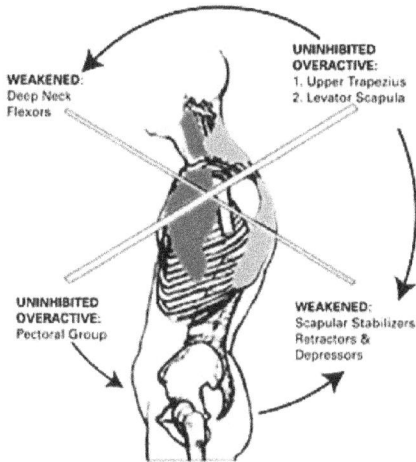

## Shoulder Blade Positioning and Posture

If you are already feeling the effects of Upper-Cross Syndrome positioning your shoulder blades can be a tough job. It can, however, be done even with imbalances present.

In a perfect world your shoulder blades would rest two inches from your spine—slightly retracted and depressed.

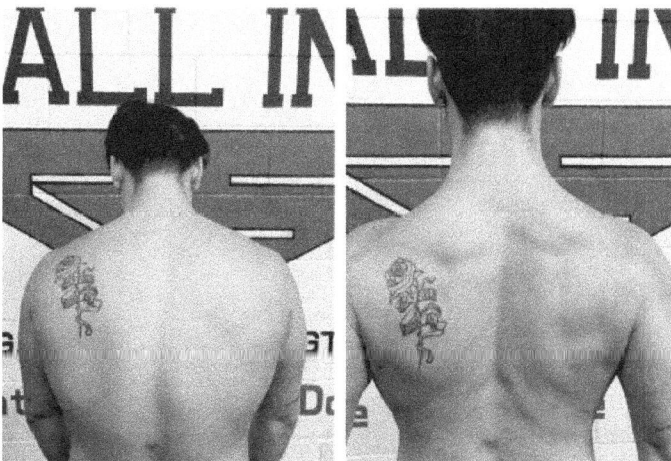

For most, this isn't the case. Some form of upper-body imbalance is present for most people—causing a misalignment of the scapulae. Being conscious of shoulder blade positioning and posture, however, can improve alignment and, subsequently, improve neutral spine position.

## Scapular Alignment

Improving the positioning of your scapulae is as simple as pulling your shoulder blades back and down. As you sit, stand, walk or train; align your shoulder blades by "putting them in your back pocket."

Consciously retracting and depressing your shoulder blades will help to make good scapular alignment possible without conscious thought. It is, however, a gentle retraction and depression.

### *Posture*

Taking conscious action to align your shoulder blades will improve your posture—there is no denying that fact. There are, however, several other great tricks for improving your posture and position of your spine.

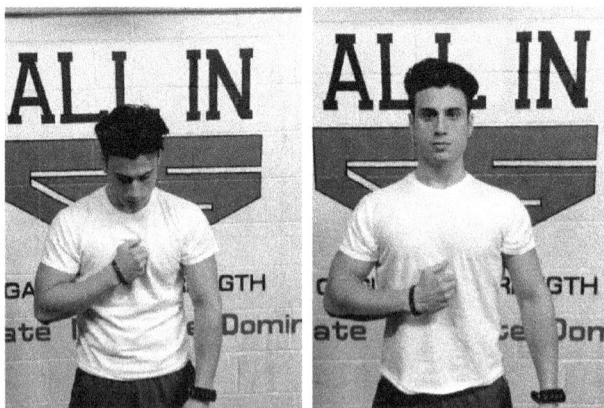

This trick takes imagination—we're sure that you have plenty. Start by pretending that there is an invisible string attached to your sternum. "Grab" the invisible string between your index finger and thumb and "pull" it. As you pull out on the string your chest should come forward and your shoulders should go back—resulting in you standing with more erect posture.

Back in the day, girls used have to walk with books on their head to reinforce good posture. Finishing school teachers would place text books on young ladies heads and have them walk around—forcing them to stand tall and erect. Pushing your head up is reminiscent of this technique.

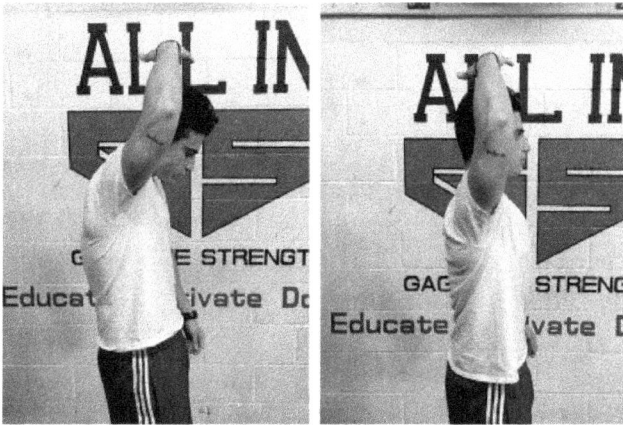

To "push your head up", place your hand on top of your head. It doesn't matter if you are seated or standing. Now use your entire body to sit erect and push the top of your head into your hand. At this point you should be sitting taller with your shoulder blades retracted, your chest out and your chin tucked.

To get the most out of these techniques, sequence them together throughout the day. Start by pulling the string and then push your head up. By really focusing on getting tall you will get in a nice neutral spine position which helps set you up for success in all of your big lifts.

## Packing the Neck

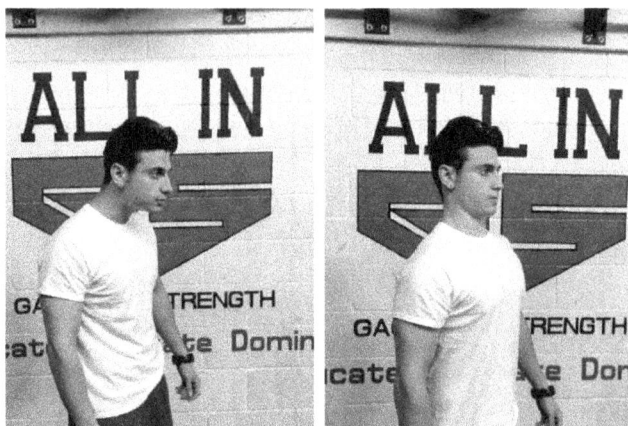

Working from the top down, neutralizing the cervical spine (neck) reinforces neutrality of the thoracic spine (upper-back) and lumbar spine (lower-back). The cervical spine is aligned in the neutral position by a technique called neck packing.

Packing the neck by pulling the chin back activates the deep cervical flexors, a group of muscles that are typically weakened by forward head posture. Unfortunately, forward head posture is common across all populations—athletic and sedentary.

Activating the deep cervical flexors not only pulls the neck into neutral alignment, but also creates stability in the cervical segment of the spine. More stability results in more strength.

The packed neck position should be held throughout all lifts—maximal or submaximal. It is also great to maintain neutral neck posture by periodically packing the neck throughout the day to activate the deep cervical flexors.

*The main key here especially during maximal lifting the neck is part of the spine and should be stable. The athlete shouldn't be looking up to much or down too much. You want the entire spine from the ears to butt to remain straight.*

*I personally like to cue my athletes to have their eyes look up when coming out of the bottom of a squat or deadlift because where the head goes the body goes. The key here is you don't want any excessive movement at the neck but the eyes can be a great driver to ensure the athlete finishes all of their grinding attempts in good position and posture.*

## Neutral Spine While Lifting

To maintain neutrality of the spine while lifting, push your chest out, then push your head up, before you brace your core. These posturing techniques will align your spine and the brace will hold it in position.

For maximal effort lifts, hold the air in your belly. This ensures the intra-abdominal pressure necessary to maintain neutral posture. You'll be safer and stronger.

Non-maximal efforts should be done without holding your breath. You'll still brace hard to maintain neutral posture, but you will breathe diaphragmatically by breathing into your belly.

When in doubt, think breathing, bracing and getting tall.

## Conclusion

Mastering the basics is like a snowball rolling down hill—the cumulative effect ends in a big result. Control your breathing, solidify your brace and create as much tension as possible. The end result will be greater stability, a neutral spine and the optimal opportunity to demonstrate strength.

# MOVEMENT PREPARATION PHASE

## Purpose and Goals

Every sound structure has a strong foundation—your body is not an exception. The Movement Preparation Phase is designed to give you the sound foundation that you need to be successful during any powerlifting program. This foundation is based on sound movement. Optimal athletic performance is centered on sound movement. As a wise man once said, you can't shoot a cannon out of a canoe.

In building our strong foundation we will achieve three goals: groove efficient movement patterns, develop general work capacity and correct muscular imbalances.

## Grooving Efficient Movement Patterns

All human movement is based on basic movement patterns—squat, hinge, push, pull and carry. Getting in and out of a chair requires a squat; picking up a pencil that you dropped takes a hinge and bringing fire wood in from outside is indubitably a carry. Throughout your day, I'm sure you also open a door at some point (pull) and replace coffee on a high shelf in a cupboard (push). These movement patterns are encompassing of daily life and integral to a successful strength and conditioning program.

Before we move on to heavy deadlifting, overhead pressing and lunge variations we have to groove the basic movement patterns. That's why this phase is called movement preparation. We are preparing your body to handle more complex versions of the basic human movements.

By the end of this phase, you should hinge like a door, squat with fluidity, and carry like a lumberjack. As a result you'll be better prepared to deadlift, barbell squat and load the bar for heavy upper-body training.

## Developing General Work Capacity

Recovery is the key to training. Irrespective of sets, reps, and volume and exercise selection—if you can't recover from the work you are doing you won't adapt to your program. Without recovery, training is destructive rather than constructive.

Gleaming at the other end of the spectrum is optimal recovery. In the optimal recovery zone our bodies become machines. The optimal recovery zone, however, is difficult to find. Recovering optimally requires a nutritional strategy, rest and a level of base fitness.

This base of fitness can also be called general physical preparedness (GPP), which the legendary Louie Simmons refers to as, "A degree of fitness that is an extension of absolute strength." For athletes, all training that isn't skill specific to their given sport is technically GPP. But the movement prep phase—with its high volume per set and short rest periods—is especially geared toward developing a general fitness level that will aid in adapting to the subsequent phases of the program.

## Correcting Muscular Imbalances

Most people walking the planet have a muscular imbalance of one form or another. Day after day people—especially athletes—move in the same patterns and hold the same postures. This causes some muscles to become short while others lengthen—limiting joint range of motion and leading to movement compensations. During this phase movements will be stripped to their most basic, restoring balance your muscles' length-tension ratios. We will also break the typical linear patterns by including movement variations in different movement planes.

## A Note for Beginners and Young Trainees

A slow and steady approach to training is most appropriate for beginners and young trainees. With that in mind, the movement prep phase can be extended to continue to master basic training skills and ensure balance throughout the body.

Beginners can extend the program phases for up to six weeks. To progress, add weight to movements, cut rest periods or add reps to movements (no more than twenty reps per set).

Young athletes can train exclusively using the movement prep program phase. Remember, for them it is about sound movement and learning to use the body. Loading them with heavy squats and deadlifts is often unnecessary. Use the progression format suggested for beginners that are extending the program.

### Keys to Success

### Picking the Right Weight

As you examine your training card, you'll see that the reps for this phase are high. This, however, doesn't mean that you will be working anywhere near failure. In fact, you should not fail during any set of this phase—as it is designed to groove good patterns. Picking a weight, however, is easy.

Coach Jim Wendler frequently talks about his starting too light philosophy. We agree with him. If you are trying an exercise for the first time—be honest with yourself and start with a weight that you know will be too light. You'll most likely get a few reps in and realize that the weight is too light—that's fine. Cut the set right there and go grab a heavier weight.

Trial and error while progressively moving up in weight is the best way to select a weight during this phase. If you're experienced, however, and know your limitations, just make sure that you pick a weight that will leave a few reps in the tank at the end of each set.

## Performing the Reps

Each rep should be smooth and controlled during this phase—moving with good form is the ultimate goal. Don't worry about how long the eccentric or concentric part of each lift is, just move with control. With that being said, don't make reps excessively long. Keep each rep under three seconds of total time under tension and you'll be in good shape.

*EXAMPLE Exercises that would be a good fit for a Movement Prep Program*

## Upper-Body

### *Push-Ups*

*What's it train?* : Upper-body pressing strength (horizontal), shoulder stability, shoulder mobility, core stability (anti-extension), muscular endurance, relative strength.

*Why use it now?* : Building shoulder and core stability, as well as shoulder mobility, will prepare you for the heavy training to come.

### *Tall Kneeling One Arm Overhead Press*

*What's it train?*   Upper-body pressing strength (vertical), shoulder mobility, shoulder stability, and core stability (anti-extension)

*Why use it now?* : It is an exercise that progresses into the barbell overhead press, a great assistance exercise to help your bench prss. Shoulder mobility and stability, as well as core stability, are important for successful and safe barbell pressing.

### *Inverted Rows*

*What's it train?* Upper-body pulling strength (horizontal), core stability, relative strength, muscular endurance

*Why use it now?* Inverted rows progress into more complex bodyweight pulling exercises. You'll learn how to effectively handle your bodyweight while building pulling strength and endurance.

## Lower-Body

### Goblet Squat

*What's it train?* : Lower-body pushing strength, squat patterning, core stability

*Why use it now?* : Goblet squats teach the squatting mechanics necessary for squatting with heavy loads. Mastering the squat pattern is important for all athletes.

### Bottoms-up Hip Thrust

*What's it train?* Hip extension, lower-body pulling strength, glute strength, and core stability

*Why use it now?* Strong glutes and powerful hip extensions improve athletic performance and prevent injury. We'll start building strong hip extension early and maintain it throughout the program.

### Dumbbell Belly Swing

*What's it train?* Hip extension (hip hinge mechanics), core stability

*Why use it now?* Good hip hinging mechanics must be mastered before barbell deadlifting or completing other advanced hip dominant movements.

## Core and Grip

### Short Lever Side Plank

*What's it train?* Core stability (anti-lateral flexion, anti-rotation), shoulder stability

*Why use it now?* Anti-lateral flexion exercises will become increasingly complex as the program progresses—short lever side planks begin the progression.

### Dead Bugs

*What's it train?* Core stability (hip flexion with neutral spine), corrects anterior pelvic tilt.

*Why use it now?* Correcting anterior pelvic tilt early in a program promotes core stability and will prepare for more complex movements during which neutral hips are necessary.

### Dumbbell Farmer's Walk

*What's it train?* Grip strength, posture, core stability (anti-rotation, anti-extension), and isometric upper-back strength.

*Why use it now?* : Farmer's walks are a great addition at any point during a program—you'll be carrying things for the rest of your life!

*Sample Movement Prep Workout*

*A1) Goblet Squat 4x8–10 reps*

*A2) Bottom Up Push Up 4x10–12 Reps*

*A3) Short Level Side Plank 4x :20 seconds*

*B1) Inverted Rows 5x10–12 reps*

*B2) Single Leg Bottom Up Hip Thrust 5x8–10 reps per side*

*B3) Deadbugs 5x 6–8 reps per side*

# POWERLIFTING NOVICE PHASES- PHASE 1

## Purpose and Goals

Smooth transitions go a long way to ensure strength and conditioning success. Each phase of a program should build upon the phase that came before it, with the adaptations blending to make you stronger, fitter and more athletic. Phase 1 is designed to help you move seamlessly from the Movement Prep Program into heavier strength training.

Before we get to the max effort work planned for phases 2 and 3, you'll need base levels of strength, hypertrophy to support your strength gains, smooth movement under tension and general work capacity. These are our goals for Phase 1.

## Base Levels of Strength

Before we train movements to max effort, we need to build a proficient level of strength with reps at mid-range intensities. Building base strength helps you get used to using heavier weights while setting the stage for greater neural adaptations from max effort training. During Phase 1 we'll take the next step in building a foundation that you could shoot a cruise missile from, forget about a cannon. Our weapons in the battle to build strength will variations of the main lifts to help build weak points and stimulate muscular growth. These movements will ingrain the motor patterns necessary for successful max effort lifts.

## Hypertrophy

We're not bodybuilders; we are athletes and strength addicts. Our biceps are just a tool in helping us pull more weight, not the focus of our training. Ed Coan once said that biceps are like ornaments on a Christmas tree.

That being said, gains in size support gains in strength—it's easier to make a bigger muscle stronger. You won't be pumping reps of biceps curls and triceps kick-backs, but by using higher volume and short rest periods you'll put enough stress on your body to make it grow.

## Smooth Movement under Tension

Developing base levels of strength and training for smooth movement under tension go hand in hand. Using sets of reps between six and eight with big movements trains you to groove good movement patterns while handling an appreciable amount of weight. You'll learn to stay tight, keep the reps consistent and move with purpose—all of which are necessary for successful max effort training.

## Building General Work Capacity

Assistance work during Phase 1 increases in volume each week while the rest periods stay relatively short (one minute). High volume training, plus short rest periods, equal a lot of oxygen intake. The training effect from this phase won't only be that of strength and size, but you'll also gain a better level of conditioning.

## Keys to Success

## Picking the Right Weight

Phase 1 introduces the concept of main lifts and accessory lifts—apples and oranges when it comes to making weight selections. Let's break things down.

Main lifts are the big, compound movements used to build strength—accessory lifts are used to improve movement, athleticism and boost subsequent performances on the main lifts. Accessory lifts are also used to increase volume for adaptations such as improved work capacity and hypertrophy. Understanding the goals of each makes weight selection easier.

The rep range for the main lifts during Phase 1 is between six and eight. If we are thinking in terms of rep maxes, your eight rep max is about eighty percent of your one rep max and your six rep max is about eighty-five percent of your one rep max. Even though we aren't necessarily working to rep maxes, these figures should give you a good idea of where to start with picking a weight. As always, starting too light is a good idea. Performing the exercise with ascending weight each set is a great strategy—in fact we recommend it.

For example if you know your 1RM in the bench press is 340 your eight rep max is probably around 275. So if were performing 3 sets of 6 you could do ascending sets or sets across.

Here's an example of ascending sets for a long pause bench:
*Set #1: 225 x 6*
*Set # 2: 250 x 6*
*Set #3: 275 x 6*

*You top set will be pretty challenging but still leaving 1-2 reps in the tank*

*Sets across might be 3 sets at 6 at 255*

All sets will be decent difficulty but you will leave a few reps left in the tank.

As you get to know your number better your ascending sets may look something like this with smaller jumps

Set #1 240x6
Set #2 255x6
Set #3 270x6

The overall volume is higher than the first example even though the top set is a little lower. You are doing more high quality work.

Let's say, hypothetically, that these are your weights for week one on the front squat. If you carry these weights over to week two, doing each for a set of eight, you will have gotten stronger and added more volume to your training. This should be your goal as you progress from week one to week two.

As you go into week three, make sure you aren't using the same weight for sets of six again—put more weight on the bar!

Choosing weights for the assistance exercises is a slightly different animal. Starting too light and working up still applies to assistance movements, but once you hit your work weight for week one you will keep it, or increase it, during the subsequent weeks. This works well because we will be increasing the volume from week to week, making your body adapt to lifting the same amount of weight more times. The end result is a bigger and stronger you.

**Performing the Reps**

Like I talked about above, exercises are broken down into main lifts and accessory lifts. The main lifts are further broken down into full range of motion and partial range of motion lifts. Accessory lifts are all done for the same volume, so there can be some continuity as to how the reps are performed. For simplicity's sake, let's break down the main lifts and accessory lifts—addressing them categorically.

*Main Lifts:*

*Full Range of Motion*

Using controlled anger is the best way to describe how to perform the full range of motion main lifts during Phase 1. During the lowering (eccentric) portion of the lift you will need to have the weight under control. I am not talking about a four second eccentric (those will come later), just make sure that the weight, or your body, isn't in a freefall. Keep the down phase around one second and you'll be doing well. On the way up you'll turn on the anger—moving the bar with as much speed  force as possible; done within the confines of good form. Pushing or pulling  the bar violently—with as much force as possible—excites your nervous  system and recruits more muscle. This is pivotal for building strength.

### Accessory Lifts:

Be smooth. It works for picking up the ladies (or gentlemen) and for successful reps during accessory lifts. One second eccentric followed by a one second concentric will do nicely. Approach each set with intensity and move fluidly. If your goal is to build more muscle adding in slower eccentrics is always an option as well to increase time under tension.

### Focusing on the Basics

*As you start to load exercises more intensely keeping the basics in mind becomes increasingly important. Focusing on bracing, setting your grip and creating tension can't be after thoughts. Make sure that your air is coming in and going to the right place—your belly. Your grip has to be intense during the big lifts. Squeeze the bar hard—as if you are trying to crush it. Create tension throughout your entire body and keep it throughout the set. If you feel yourself losing tension, pause and reset before doing the next rep.*

*If you need a refresher, check "Mastering the Basics" at the beginning of this handbook.*

*Here are some sample exercises that would be used during a building phase*

### Upper-Body

### Wide Grip Feet  - Up Press with long pause

*What's it train?* : Horizontal upper-body pressing strength

*Why use it now?* : Feet up pressing is great for developing pushing strength since it teacher you the proper groove and how to utilize your chest when benching. Your legs are also taken out of the equation—allowing you to focus on positioning your upper-body and elbows correctly without worrying about your legs.

### Z-Press

*What's it train?* : Vertical upper-body pressing strength, core stability

*Why use it now?* : The Z-Press builds a serious amount of core stability while working on pressing strength. Sitting upright on the floor also controls the amount of weight you can press—limiting the stress on your shoulders and Central Nervous System early in the program. You'll build a strong foundation to improve your standing overhead press. This exercise will also ingrain overhead pressing mechanics because you are forced to stay upright. Unless you stay tall, and stay in your pressing groove, you won't be able to use any appreciable weight.

### Rack Row

*What's it train?* Upper-body pulling strength, grip strength, isometric posterior chain strength, and hip positioning/neutral spine

*Why use it now?* Rack rows begin the progression into doing full-range bent row variations. Starting with a partial range of motion makes it easier to learn to pull heavy weight while keeping the hips in a good position with the spine neutral. Bent row variations have tremendous carry-over to the deadlift because they tax the entire posterior chain.

## Lower-Body

## Front Squat

*What's it train?* Lower-body pushing strength, core stability, and upper-back isometric strength

*Why use it now?* Front squats are a great next step after the goblet squats used in the movement prep phase. Not only are they great for improving strength in the lower-body, but they also improve squat patterning, core strength, and upper-back strength. This one lift improves athleticism and has carry-over to both the squat and the deadlift.

## Double Overhand Low Rack Pull

*What's it train?* Lower-body pulling strength, hip hinge mechanics, core stability, upper-back strength, and grip strength

*Why use it now?* Partial range of motion deadlifts improve performance on full-range deadlifts by teaching good form and proper recruitment sequencing. When used in a submaximal repetition format they can build full-body mass. The double overhand grip helps train grip strength and limits the stress on the central nervous system.

## Romanian Deadlift (RDL)

*What's it train?* Lower-body pulling strength, hip hinge mechanics, core stability, upper-back strength, grip strength

*Why use it now?* RDL is a classic exercise used to develop the posterior chain. It is great for prepping the hamstrings

## Core and Grip

## Unilateral Farmer's Walk

*What's it train?* Core stability (anti-lateral flexion, anti-rotation) and grip

*Why use it now?* Unilateral farmer's walks are great for beginning the progression into heavier asymmetrically loaded core training. The movement under tension helps to build upon your level of general physical preparedness.

## Plank Walk Back

*What's it train?* Core stability (anti-extension), shoulder stability

*Why use it now?* Plank walk backs are the moving version of a superman plank (an exercise you'll be doing in a later phase of the program). Moving in and out of the superman plank position is easier than holding the position statically—thus plank walk backs begin the progression to the superman plank.

## Landmines

*What's it train?* Core stability (anti-rotation, anti-extension), shoulder stability

*Why use it now?* The heavy squatting and deadlifting you'll do in later phases of the program will require serious levels of core stability—requiring us to build a lot of core stability now. Landmines train the core in the standing position which has important carry-over to squatting, deadlifting, overhead pressing, and sports.

### Sample Building Phase Workout Squat Focused

*A1) Front Squat 4x6*

*B1) RDL 3x8*

*C1) Unilateral Farmers Walk 3x:30 seconds per side*

*C2) Bulgarian Split Squat 3x10 per side*

*C3) Band Side Steps 2x20 per side*

# POWERLIFTING INTERMEDIATE PHASES - PHASE 2

Accomplishing your Phase 1 goals has taken you one step closer to hitting new PRs. But it's not time to get comfortable—there's no such thing as satisfied.

During Phase 2, we'll take things to the next level by introducing Westside Conjugate Method (WCM) training. Two days per week will be devoted to max effort training, while two more will be devoted to dynamic effort training. Focusing on these two methods you'll build starting strength, better rate of force development and prepare to peak.

## Starting Strength

Our first goal shares its name with a popular training book by Mark Rippetoe and Lon Kilgore. While Rippetoe and Kilgore describe the basic barbell lifts and how to perform them in their book, we are talking more about building maximal concentric strength out of mid-point to bottom position of two big lifts—the squat and the bench press. We are going to build a strong push while limiting the amount of eccentric stress. This trains the nervous system while limiting muscle damage—making you stronger and allowing for great recovery.

Learning to move maximal weights during concentric only lifts is great preparation for full range of motion max effort training. It allows for movement mastery with the absence of eccentric training stress.

We'll use our assistance lifts to build strength and movement proficiency. They'll keep your body in balance as you build greater levels of strength.

## Rate of Force Development

How quickly can you display speed and power? Good sport coaches will ask every team sport athlete this question. The dynamic effort days during Phase 2 will be concentrated on developing high levels of rate of force development—helping you to put more weight on the bar during your max effort training and move powerfully as an athlete. Power is the key to transferring maximal strength to athletic performance. You are about to become a powerhouse.

Dave Tate likens rate of force development to punching through glass. If you really want to break the window you won't press on it slowly and progressively generate more force—you'll throw your fist at the glass as quickly as possible. Consider the glass your sticking point on a given lift and your fist, rate of force development. Remember, speed kills but power punishes!

## Preparing to Peak

Phase 2 is a rung in the ladder leading to the ultimate peak at the end of Phase 3. Phase 2 by itself will make you stronger and more powerful, but it is also designed to prepare your body for the volume and intensity of Phase 3. At its essence, Phase 2 was constructed to transition you from the base strength built during Phase 1 and the maximal strength development of Phase 3.

## Keys to Success

## Picking the Right Weight

WCM includes several different loading parameters—max effort method (concentric only), dynamic effort method and repetition effort method. All three of these parameters will be included during Phase 2 programming; and all three will require different weight selection processes.

## Max Effort Method *(main lift variations only)*:

If you aren't used to this form of training—picking a weight can be a challenge. We suggest using ascending sets.

By using ascending sets. you'll simply progress up to work sets by adding more weight to the bar each time you lift it. Work up to a weight that rates between nine and ten on your personal rate of perceived exertion scale. Once you've done this, look at the weights that you used for your previous sets—if they are ninety percent of your hardest set they count toward your total sets for the day. If you don't have enough total sets at or above ninety percent, go back down to ninety percent (or a little above) of the heaviest weight you used and finish your sets.

## Max Effort Method *(full range)*:

Picking the weights for the full-range lifts is similar to choosing weights for the variations of the lifts. The difference is you probably have a better idea of what you can do through a full range of motion. You'll still use an ascending set up, but consult a rep max chart as a guide in choosing weights for your sets. As an example, your three rep max is about ninety to ninety-three percent of your one rep max.

## Dynamic Effort Method:

Picking a weight for your dynamic effort exercises will be easy as usually the percent is set already in a program. These weights, however, are not set in stone.

Your main concern should be with bar speed. If the bar is moving slow at the weight we've prescribed, then you need to reduce the bar weight until are moving with better speed. Likewise, if you feel as though you can move fast with a little bit more weight on the bar—please do so. As a caution, be sure not to get overzealous if you increase the weight above the prescribed percentage. If there is even a hint that the bar speed might slow down drop the weight back down.

A big idea here is to start around 50% of your max and go from there.

If you are using a lot of chain weight or band tension in general use less bar weight. If you are using straight weight a higher percentage must be used.

## Performing the Reps

Maximal force and maximal speed are the two biggest keys to successfully performing reps using the WCM. Even though the bar may move slowly, while training with the max effort method, your focus should still be on moving the bar as fast as possible. You'll do the same for the dynamic effort method—pushing and pulling with maximal force and maximal speed.

It's important to avoid failing on a lift during your max effort training, as this can wreak havoc on your nervous system. If you do miss a lift, however, you must account for it as two completed sets and cut the rest of your volume down. For example, if you fail during your fourth set of Anderson Half Squats you need to count that as two sets—eliminating your fifth set. For the sixth set you will drop down to a manageable weight and concentrate on moving with good form and speed. This applies to all max effort training during phases 2 and 3. Push yourself, but be smart about it.

Approach the repetition effort training with the same mentality—especially as the set wears on and fatigue starts to set in. The goal is to be powerful even when you're tired.

Dominating your repetition effort training by generating as much power as possible up to the last rep will train you to be powerful in the face of fatigue. Just like in sports, you should always be in a good position—even if you are tired.

We'll keep the same rules for the accessory lifts. Be smooth. One second extra,followed by a one second concentric will do nicely. Approach each set with intensity and move fluidly.

## Focusing on the Basics

As the weights get bigger the little things become more important. Attack each rep of every set with focus—solidifying your bracing technique, controlling your air, and creating as much tension possible.

If you need a refresher, check "Mastering the Basics" at the beginning of the manual.

*Sample Strength Phase Exercises*

## Upper-Body

### Standing Overhead Press with pause

*What's it train?* Maximal vertical upper-body pressing strength, upper-back strength, and core stability

*Why use it now?* Performing the overhead press now in a heavy three rep format will prepare you for the heavy singles programmed for this exercise during Phase 3 and during testing.

### Speed Bench Press

*What's it train?* Horizontal upper-body pressing strength and power, rate of force development starting strength

*Why use it now?* Rate of force development is important for improving maximal strength and athletic performance. Dynamic effort training started now will prepare you to peak during testing and perform during your competitive season.

### Mid-Point Pin Press

*What's it train?* Maximal horizontal upper-body pressing strength starting strength

*Why use it now?* The mid-point pin press builds starting strength, a main goal for Phase 2. This exercise will help to build chest, triceps, and shoulder strength that bolsters performance on the overhead press.

## Lower-Body

## Anderson Half Squat

*What's it train?* Maximal lower-body pushing strength (concentric only), starting strength, and core stability

*Why use it now?* Anderson Half Squats build starting strength and teach your body to generate force without pre-stretching the muscles. You'll progress up to paused squats in Phase 3. Half squats will prepare you for them.

## Conventional Speed Deadlifts

*What's it train?* Lower-body pulling strength and power, rate of force development, core stability, and grip strength

*Why use it now?* Conventional speed deadlifts are a great introduction to the dynamic effort method of training because of their small learning curve. They develop powerful hip extension that carries over to your weight-room performance and athletic performance.

## Dynamic Effort Squats

*What's it train?* Lower-body strength and power, rate of force development, core stability

*Why use it now?* Dynamic builds serious lower-body power. Dynamic work will help dial in your technique and speed with the squat pattern.

**Assistance Moves**

**Barbell Glute Bridge**

*What's it train?* Hip extension strength and core stability

*Why use it now?* Barbell glute bridges build serious hip extension strength by teaching the glutes to move weight. Strong, glute dominant hip extension is important for the overall health of your body and athletic performance.

**One Arm Dumbbell Row**

*What's it train?* : Horizontal upper-body pulling strength (unilateral), core stability, grip strength

*Why use it now?* : Unilateral pulling strength is important for the health of your upper-back and shoulders. Pulling unilaterally also supports core stability.

**Bar Rollouts**

*What's it train?* Core stability (anti-extension), lat strength, and extensibility

*Why use it now?* Bar rollouts are a progress from the planking variations used during the Movement Prep Phase and Phase 1.

**Sample Strength Phase 2 Workout Dynamic Effort**

A1) Box Squat with chains 10x2 at 60%

B1) Speed Deadlift 6x1 at 70%

C1) Bar Roll out  3x10

C2) Barbell Glute Bridge 3x8

## POWERLIFTING PEAKING PHASES- PHASE 3

### Purpose and Goals

Up until now, you've improved your movement quality, built a base of strength, and cut your gums on the WCM. Now it's time to attack Phase 3—as it culminates in the development of absolute strength. But first, you have one month full of ass busting training. Intensity is the theme of Phase 3.

Conjugate training will be in full swing during Phase 3 with full range max effort training and increased volume dynamic effort training. Every exercise—from core training to deadlifting—is designed to give your body the stimuli it needs to reach peak performance. This means that there is only one goal for Phase 3—achieve a new PR.

### Pursuing New PRs

What does it mean to achieve new goals and how will you know if you've done it?

At the onset of the program, after you tested, I told you to write down your goals for each of the test lifts and put them somewhere you would see them every day. In doing this, we wanted you to make an emotional attachment to your goals. Committing to facing your goals every day gives you the positive mental imagery and focus necessary to achieve greatness.

Achieving a new personal record is just like about attaining greatness in your life. Hitting a new PR is the realization that you did everything you could to make yourself better during a program—and having the results to prove it.

At the end of a peaking Phase 3 you will test, you will conquer the goals you set out for yourself and you will now have new goals to strive for.

**Keys to Success**

**Picking the Right Weight**

Phase 3 continues on with WCM style training—meaning that there we will continue to use the same loading parameters as Phase 2: max effort, dynamic effort, submaximal effort and repetition effort. We've made some slight alterations, though.

*Max Effort Method*:

Your max effort exercises will all be done through a full-range of motion during Phase 3—and the percentages you will be working at are programmed. The guess work for picking weights is done for you, just don't get over zealous. If you are off your game, and the bar alone feels like a ton, cut your losses and work at a lower percentage or move on to your assistance work.

If you feel great, however, feel free to pile on the weight. The goal is to strain to
overcome sticking points, both mentally and physically. Maintain your form and avoid
failing at any set.

The week before you want to test your singles, I suggest using some overload training. By using reverse bands and sling shots, you can actually feel your goal weights in your hands or on your back. This will give you the central nervous system stimulation you need to handle big weights as well as boost your confidence knowing that you already handled that number in some form already. You have seen it and conquered it.

## Dynamic Effort Method:

Your main concern should be with bar speed. If the bar is moving slowly at the weight we've prescribed, then you need to reduce the bar weight until you are moving with better speed. Likewise, if you feel as though you can move fast with a little bit more weight on the bar—please do so.

However, use caution - be sure not to get overzealous if you increase the weight above the prescribed percentage. If there is even a hint that the bar speed might slow down, drop the weight back down.

### *Submaximal Effort Method*:

As in previous phases, all of the assistance work is programmed using the submaximal effort method. For each assistance movement, pick a weight that is going to make you work but leaves a little gas in the tank. Phase 3 is the exception. If you want to push your limits during the last set of each assistance exercise during Phase 3—get after it! Again it's a good idea to pick exercises during this phase that directly hammers a weak area.

## Performing the Reps

Maximal force and maximal speed are the two biggest keys to performing successful reps using the WCM. Even though the bar may move slowly while training with the max effort method, your focus should still be on moving the bar with maximal speed. Remember, it's the intent to move the weight quickly that's most important. You'll do the same for the dynamic effort method—pushing and pulling with maximal force and maximal speed.

Approach the repetition effort training with the same mentality—especially as the set wears on and fatigue starts to set in. The goal is to be powerful even when you're tired. Dominating your repetition effort training by generating as much power as possible up to the last rep will train you to be powerful in the face of fatigue.

We'll keep the same rules for the accessory lifts. Be smooth. One second eccentric followed by a one second concentric will do nicely. Approach each set with intensity and move fluidly.

## Focusing on the Basics

As the weights get bigger the little things become more important. Attack each rep of every set with focus—solidifying your bracing technique, controlling your air and creating as much tension possible.

If you need a refresher, check "Mastering the Basics" at the beginning of the manual.

## Sample Exercises to Peaking Phase

### Sling Shot Pause Bench

*What's it train?* Overload Maximal horizontal pressing strength (with limited stretch reflex).

*Why use it now?* Benching with a sling shot will allow you to overload your bench so you can feel heavier weights in your hands, which is critical for preparing you to test your competition bench press.

## Reverse Band Squat

*What's it train?* Maximal lower-body pushing strength with overload, upper-back strength, core stability

Why use it now? : Reverse Band squats build maximal systemic strength that will carry over to your performance when testing your squat. It will allow you to feel maximal weight on your back while de-loading your position in the bottom of the movement.

## Deadlift

*What's it train?* Maximal lower-body pulling strength, back strength, core stability, and grip strength

*Why use it now?* You will be testing the deadlift at the end of Phase 3. Performing heavy singles with this lift develops maximal pulling strength and prepares you to peak for testing.

*Sample overload protocols for peaking phase*

**Squat**

*Squatting works up to around an opener (about 90%) then add reverse mini band for 2nd attempt and reverse monster mini band for 3rd attempt*

**Bench**

*Works up to around an opener (about 92.5 %) then add loose blue reactive sling shot for 2nd attempt and tight blue reactive sling shot for 3rd attempt.*

# BEYOND THE POWERLIFTING HANDBOOK

## Athletes

If you are a competitive athlete and you are utilizing this methods during your off season you're prepared to start your season with new levels of strength and athleticism—accompanied by injury resistance. But training for strength doesn't cease in the off-season—you need to keep lifting.

Lifting during the season is focused on maintaining strength—keep the volume low, limit extra stress, and keep workouts short. How often you lift depends on total volume of training, including practice, conditioning and competition. The more you practice, condition and compete the less you will lift, and vice versa.

## Strength Coaches/Lifters

We know the question in your mind, "Great! I finished this book, now what do I do?"

If you are a strength coach or lifter using this book to make your own programs better I suggest you take a look your own programs and see what lines up with The Powerlifting Handbook and what doesn't. Are you utilizing all of the methods and principles? Are you using them at the appropriate times? Are you focused on teaching the basics? Use the old adage from Bruce Lee "Adapt what is useful, reject what is useless, and add what is specifically your own."

Add in the methods and principles that fit the needs of the population you are working with.

## The Next Step

The hardest person to coach is yourself. Coaches need coaches, too! Beginners and elite athletes both need guidance. If you are unsure on how to implement these principles on your own keep on reading!

There are special offers at the very end of this book that will allow you to work directly with the team at Gaglione Strength to ensure you can become the strongest version of yourself!

Our goal is to make sure you reach yours. We are 100% committed to your success and will do whatever we can to help you out!

## SPECIAL OFFER FOR ANY STRENGTH COACHES OR GYM OWNERS

I have done many speaking engagements at various schools, universities, colleges and gym throughout the Northeast of the United States.

If you would like an in - depth review of the Powerlifting Handbook LIVE in person, our team does offers staff training and seminars. All you need to do is e-mail gaglionestrength@gmail.com with the subject line " the Powerlifting Handbook Seminar Request"

You will learn how to implement the Powerlifting Handbook principles into the current training program that you are already running. Contact us today!

# WORKS CITED

1. Hoff, J., Helgerud, J., & Wisloff, U. (1999). Maximal strength training improves work economy in trained female cross-country skiers. *Med. Sci. Sports Exerc*, *31*(6), 870-877.

2. Simmons, L. (2004). Training methods part 1: speed day. Westside Barbell. Retrieved November 29, 2011, from http://www.westside-barbell.com

3. Simmons, L. (2009). Max effort method. Westside Barbell. Retrieved November 29, 2011, from http://www.westside-barbell.com

4. Wisloff, U., Castagna, C., Hlegerud, J., Jones, R., & Hoff, J. (2004). Strong correlation of maximal squat strength with sprint. *Br J of Sports Med*, *38*, 285-288.

## TESTIMONIALS

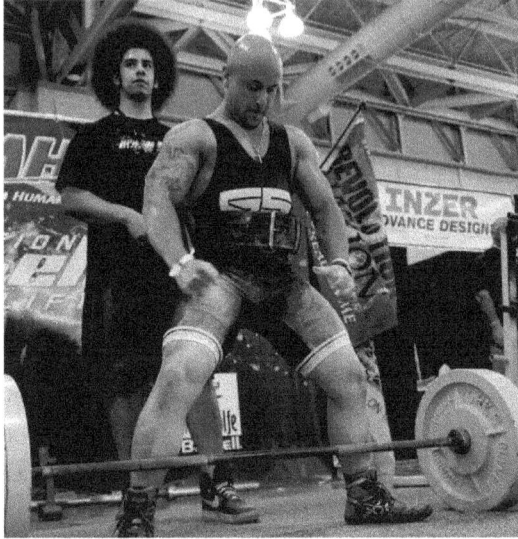

I first met John Gaglione in June 2014 at a local firness expo. Before meeting John I was just a regular guy going to the gym to be "fit." The sport of powerlifting did not exist to me as I was Naive. At this expo I won the squatting contest which awarded me a free month to try his gym, Gaglione Strength. This opportunity changed my life. John has showed me the world of powerlifting and since has become much more than a coach to me, but a mentor and a great freind.

As far as the gym aspect is concerned, John has transformed me from just a guy at the gym to a top level athlete. When we met I was squatting 315, benching 225, and deadlifting 405. In just over a year I now squat and deadlift over 500 and bench over 300. Following John's programming (mainly his meet peaking cycle) I have achieved a top 10 position in the national rankings and have a goal of soon becoming one of the best in the world.

*—Andrew Petti Nationally Ranked in the 148 Raw*
*with Wraps division*

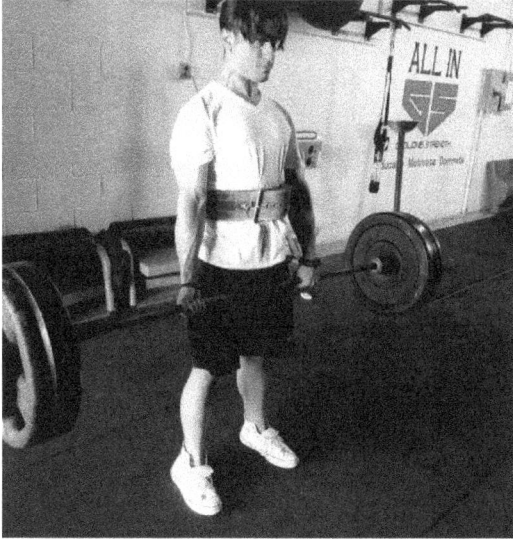

I was a personal trainer when I first met John and thought I already had a good handle on my own training. I'm a small guy who on a good day could probably pull 305 on the deadlift at the time. In 6 months John put over 100lbs on my deadlift which still amazes me how that's even possible.

—*James Posillico Strength Coach*

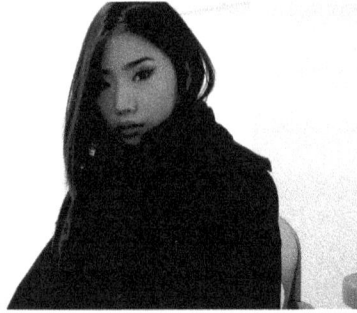

I'm grateful to be part of the team where a community exists with constant warmth and growth. I was starting to get into powerlifting and in order to train smart and safe I looked into training in Gaglione Strength. I felt uneasy about trying it out in the beginning but after the first session I fit right in. Not only my training so far has been successful with lots of PRs and getting myself out of my comfort zone, I've become rich in happiness and health as coach takes care of each individual by giving us tips and motivations on daily basis despite being occupied with other work and errands. I realize the relationship with the team that John creates is far more precious than the relationship with me and my PRs.

Current PRs:
Squat: 3RM 200
Deadlift: 3RM 240 1RM 275

—*Haemee Dai Nationally Ranked 105 Powerlifter*

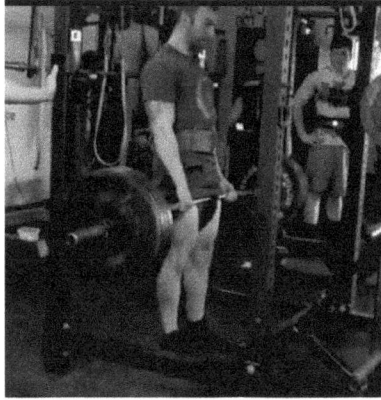

I heard about Gaglione strength and powerlifting back in March of 2015 from one of the members at my old gym. They had just told me they have competed in their first powerlifting meet and were hooked from there on out. I'm always trying find new ways to Innovate my training and challenge my self while having fun and staying safe, so hearing about this couldn't have happened at a better time. From the moment I signed up, I have seen nothing but consistent progress in both my lifts and my physique. Before coming to Gaglione strength, my squat was 335 on a good day and my deadlift was 365. Working with John and the other coaches I decided to do my first powerlifting meet in June of 2015 and got bit by the powerlifting bug, and John helped me achieve one of my first meet goals of breaking 1000lb total with a 385 squat 275 bench and 450 deadlift. Now coming up to almost a year at Gaglione Strength, I squat 435lbs and deadlift 455lbs putting close to 100lbs on both my squat and deadlift from when I started while achieving a much leaner physique and just overall gaining more confidence in myself as a person. But the best part is not only the progress you see in yourself, but the way a group of people can come together, motivate and inspire each other to push past your limits to achieve more and create such a positive environment, and that's exactly what powerlifting has to offer.

*—Nick Vogelsang - Light Weight Raw Powerlifter*

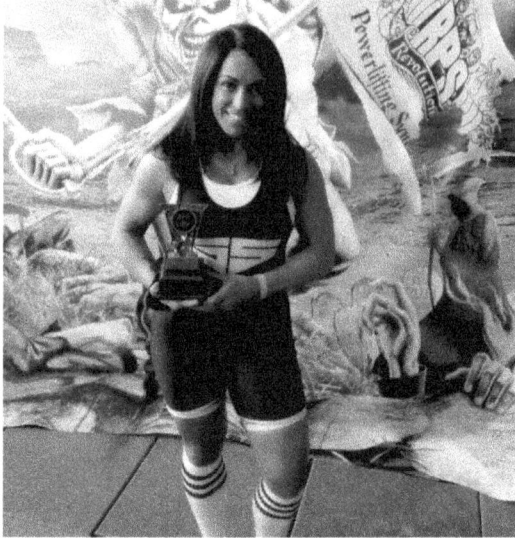

If someone would have told me that in only one year of training with coach Gaglione that I would place on the national ranking list for squat in my weight class , that I'd be benching 170 pounds for reps and deadlifting 320 pounds , I'd say they were delusional!  But here I am after only one year of following coach Gaglione's  powerlifting program and my progress has been remarkable.  Although I have always been into fitness and have done weight training  in the past for many years I, like most females have never done any sort of bench pressing and had no idea how to deadlift with proper form.  When I decided to start powerlifting I was 39 years old and it was important for me to be able to do a program that wouldn't leave me strapped to a wheel chair each week.  I found his programming to be very suitable in the fact that it gradually progressed my strength each cycle without leaving me feeling completely wiped out and hurting.  I believe that my great  progress can be attributed to the fact that I am completely dedicated to training and following coach Gaglione's program. I am looking forward to continuing powerlifting and anxious to see what the future holds for me in this sport !

*—Laura Paul - Nationally Ranked 148 Lb Raw Powerlifter  with a Current PR 345 lb Squat*

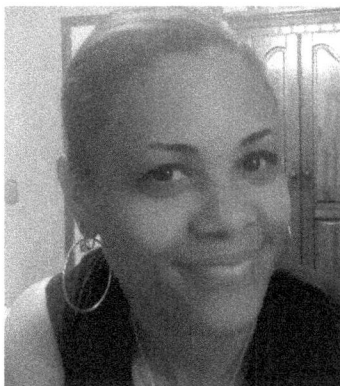

I have been weight training for about 7 years, have a background as a personal trainer, and at one time an aspiring strength and conditioning coach, and I can say without a doubt that the last year training with John has been the best I've ever had as a lifter. I've had problems squatting for most of my years lifting, and within a year John has coached me to a 300 lb squat. I can't express how unbelievable that is to me. I've never completely entrusted my programming and training to another person before and I can say without a doubt that my trust is well placed. I eagerly look forward to what the future holds for my powerlifting career and I cannot give enough thanks to John Gaglione.

*—Courtney Bumford  165 Raw Powerlifter*
*with Current PR 400 lb Deadlift*

## ABOUT THE AUTHOR

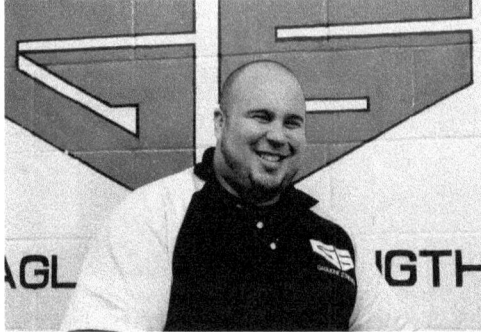

John Gaglione is a strength coach based out of Long Island, New York. John trains people from all walks of life at his facility, which is located in Farmingdale, New York. He specializes in improving maximal strength for both athletes and "average Joes" alike. John coaches a powerlifting team that consists of more than 40 lifters; over 20 of those lifters hold national ranking in their respective weight classes and divisions.

John has written many strength and conditioning articles for major online publications, such as *Men's Health, Elite Fitness Systems, Testosterone Nation, and One Result.* He is the featured strength & conditioning author for the book <u>Long Island Wrestling Association</u>. John has been a featured speaker at several schools, including Cortland and Hofstra Universities – for their exercise science programs.

As an avid strength athlete, John also has a lot of "under the bar experience," and he has competed in the sport of powerlifting for over a decade. He has the best competition lifts: an 900 Squat, 575 Bench, and a 640 Deadlift.

If you would like to learn more about John, you can reach him at **gaglionestrength@gmail.com.**

## Train with Gaglione Strength

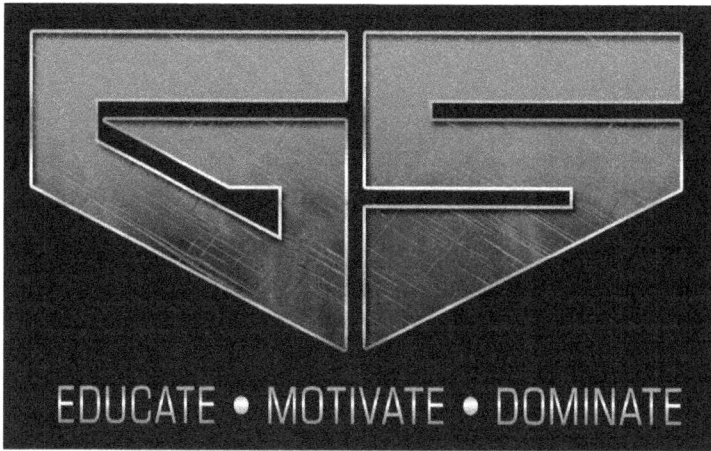

EDUCATE • MOTIVATE • DOMINATE

For locals, you can request a complimentary session and consultation by sending an e-mail to gaglionestrength@gmail.com with the subject line "Powerlifitng Handbook" and we will get your scheduled for your session.

For those who are not in the Tri-state area, you can take full advantage of our Elite Distance Coaching program by going to sending an e-mail to gaglionestrength@gmail.com with the subject line "Online Coaching Powerlifting Handbook" for a special discounted rate exclusive only to our readers.

If are a beginner or a seasoned veteran in the sport, we can help you! Our most accomplished lifter Mark Greenstein, who, at the time of this book, is ranked 5th best all time in the world in the sport of powerlifting in the 198 class with an 1825 total.

No matter where you are or what level you are at we can help you get to the next one and help you become the strongest version of you!

Whether you are just starting our or you are already elite we can help you! Don't be shy and contact us today with any questions you may have! We wish you luck on your journey to become a stronger you!

www.ingramcontent.com/pod-product-compliance
Lightning Source LLC
Chambersburg PA
CBHW020007290326

41935CB00007B/333